I0113829

BEAUTY
AT YOUR
FINGERTIPS!

Kitchen Remedies for Your Skin & Hair

Dr Nirmala Shetty is the founder of Nirmal Herbal, a successful enterprise that promotes healthy and beautiful skin and hair through the use of natural, chemical-free products. After opening a flourishing first centre in Chembur, she now has branches in Bandra, Powai, Mulund and Vile Parle.

Dr Shetty served as a beauty consultant at the Hyatt Regency in 2002. She has also officially attended to the Miss India International and Miss India World contestants, and has trained them in the use of natural beauty items. In addition, she has worked closely with former Miss Universe, Sushmita Sen, and has been the official hair expert on the panel of the 'I Am She Miss India Universe Pageant'.

Dr Shetty's participation in the serial, Beauty Mantra, with Lisa Ray, which was telecast in USA and the UK, earned wide critical acclaim. Her articles have appeared in *UpperCrust*, *Style Speak*, *Femina*, *The Bombay Times*, *The Indian Express*, and *Mid-Day*.

Dr Shetty has completed a variety of courses in naturopathy and alternative medicine, and is a certified health coach from the Institute of Integrative Nutrition, New York, USA.

BEAUTY
AT YOUR
FINGERTIPS!

Kitchen Remedies for Your Skin & Hair

DR NIRMALA SHETTY

westland ltd

61, Silverline Building, 2nd Floor, Alapakkam Main Road, Maduravoyal, Chennai 600 095

No. 38/10 (New No.5), Raghava Nagar, New Timber Yard Layout, Bengaluru 560 026

93, 1st Floor, Sham Lal Road, Daryaganj, New Delhi 110002

First published by westland ltd 2014

Copyright © Nirmala Shetty 2014

All rights reserved

10 9 8 7 6 5 4 3 2 1

ISBN: 978-93-84030-43-8

Design: seema sethi {design}

The contents of this book are for informational purposes only. Consult your doctor before beginning any new diet or beauty regimen. The author and publishers assume no responsibility for injuries suffered while following the guidelines listed in this book.

This book is sold subject to the condition that it shall not by way of trade or otherwise, be lent, resold, hired out, circulated, and no reproduction in any form, in whole or in part (except for brief quotations in critical articles or reviews) may be made without written permission of the publishers.

Contents

Foreword by Sushmita Sen   *vii*

Introduction   *ix*

Food for Thought   1

General Notes Regarding Natural Recipes   7

The Wonders of Common Kitchen Ingredients   9

Skin Care   47

    Common Skin Problems   52
    Acne, Pigmentation, Rosacea, Dark Circles

    Lip care   67

    Back care   70

Hair Care   75

    Common Hair Problems   79
    Premature Greying, Dandruff, Alopecia

Beauty & Seasons   93

    Spring   94

    Summer   104

    Monsoon   118

    Winter   127

Beauty & Age   139

    Infancy   139

    Childhood   142

    Adolescence   153

    The Prime of Life   159

Beauty & the Man   167

Beauty & Weddings   173

    Post-Engagement   175

    The Month Before the Wedding   179

    The Wedding   181

Case Studies & Testimonials   185

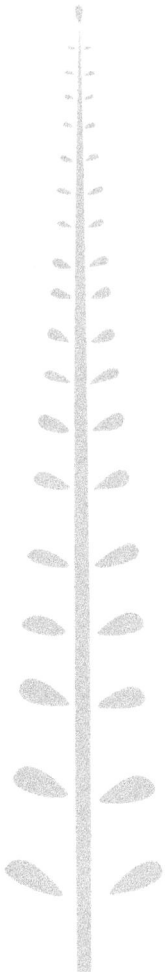

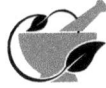

Foreword

If I had but one principle to live by, it would be to live in accordance with the laws of nature.

They are made by God – the label reads 'Made in Heaven'. And I love all things heavenly and godly!

I have great regard for the cures, treatments and recipes that come from the kitchens of our mothers and grandmothers – kitchens that are full of love and natural herbs and spices. And a love that has withstood the test of time and doles out care and cures in rhythm with the wisdom of the cosmos.

Even today, I use tips given by my mother and my mother's mother, collected over the years, and carried forward by Renee and Alisah – the gen-next mothers-in-line!

A little habit cultivated daily goes a long way towards nurturing ourselves. For instance, brushing and flossing our teeth keeps our original set intact a hundred years hence. I, till date, pamper my skin morning and evening, cleaning, toning, moisturising, come what may.

My vision for our world is simple – on earth as it is in heaven. All we need are people who believe, and people who act on that belief. Dr Nirmala Shetty is a great example of such a person.

I thank her profusely for taking under her wing 70 young women contestants from all 3 pageants of 'I AM She Miss Universe India'. For teaching them and showing them how to make their hair and skin glow from within – the hallmark of real beauty.

Open up… apply… and blossom!

Dr Nirmala Shetty is a name I love and trust! The very best to her always.

Sushmita Sen
Actor and Former Miss Universe

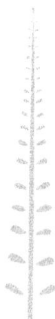

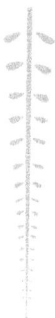

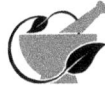

Introduction

All of us are born beautiful

Mothers across the world have loved their babies and cherished them, nurtured them as the most precious of beings. Yet sadly, such careful fostering can come to naught. As the little child grows, and is exposed to the media, or to harsh peer groups, she starts feeling self-conscious. What if she isn't as fine-looking as her mother claimed she was? What if she does not match society's norms of beauty?

Which brings me to a pertinent question: What are these norms?

Well, in India, the first median of attractiveness is the fairest possible skin colour. This is odd, since even a rudimentary study of science and anthropology will tell us that our skin colour is directly linked to the part of the globe we hail from, and the genes we inherit.

Furthermore, Nature herself loves colour, all colours; this is obvious when we soak in the diversity around us, observe plants, birds and animals. If we can accept myriad hues in general, why is it hard for us to acknowledge that every human being has a colour that is different?

The multiplicity of skin colours, and the beauty of all tones is a concept I wish to emphasise, for I know millions of

Indians who would go to absurd lengths to become fair. The fault, to some extent, lies with the society we live in, where potential mothers-in-law will only let their sons marry a fair bride, or bashful grooms insist on wives with 'wheatish' skin. Never mind if the boy himself is dark complexioned or the mother-in-law is a rich dark brown! I have yet to find a matrimonial column that says: 'Wanted: A bride with healthy skin'. Such a pity!

The truth is, the dark skinned are fortunate! Those with dusky complexions have more melanin than their fairer counterparts. This melanin protects them, allows them to withstand the heat of the sun, fight skin disorders, and even combat the ageing process. Fair skinned people on the other hand have a fair share of trouble! They get tanned easily, sunburnt, have pigmentation problems and discoloured skin. Now that's a handful.

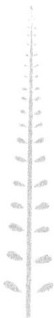

x

We need to remember that when people state that black is beautiful, they aren't referring merely to clothes, shoes and purses. They are referring to the fortunate men and women who are dusky and gorgeous.

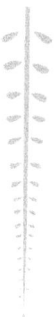

A second median of beauty in India and across the world is flawless skin – a skin free of acne, blemishes, and dullness. The quality of skin is linked to one's internal and external health; skin ailments are conditions created by the body itself. Luckily, I have some remedies that I will be discussing with you in the chapters that follow.

The third median of beauty is hair. While everyone may yearn for thick tresses, each of us is born with a definite number of hair follicles; this varies from person to person, and determines the thickness of his or her hair. The growth, length, colour, and lustre of our hair depends on the usual suspects – the genetic pool, internal and external health, and lifestyle choices.

As we see, socially-imposed norms of beauty are flawed, for they fail to acknowledge the diversity and the magnificent multiplicity of the human race.

Ignoring societal expectations, what we can do is ensure that our skin and hair is healthy. It has been my vision to make every skin type glow flawlessly without chemicals, without makeup, and make every type of hair grow lustrously. In both cases, I depend on the things we find in our kitchen. The food we eat to live is the food I use to treat skin and hair. The memories of my grandmother's recipes from the kitchen are brought alive each time I approach an ailment or complaint.

Nature is filled with magic in abundance. We are gifted with the purest vitamins, minerals and nutrients in the form of fruits, vegetables, herbs and dry fruits. It is for this reason that I insist that one must dip into something natural for the skin and hair at least once or twice a day. Moreover, what we apply on our bodies is ingested by it. The cream that causes a rash, the talc that irritates, all of these find a way into our bodies. If this be the case, don't you think it's necessary to make sure that the products you apply are safe and healthy? And what could be better that fruits, vegetables and herbs?

Ancient history bears witness to ageless beauty acquired with natural products like milk, sandalwood and almonds. Remember Cleopatra who bathed in ass' milk? Nature has been exploited for beauty products, be it today or in the distant past. In our day and age, of course, time and energy may not permit us to grind spices and make beauty potions daily. But the least one can do is utilise simple and plentifully available ingredients like milk, curd, honey, tomatoes, and cucumbers to maintain the skin and hair. Today, image management plays a vital role in every field of work from front office desk jobs and airline posts,

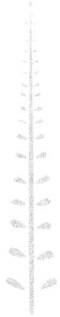

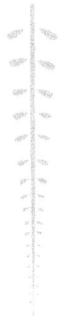

to modelling, acting or anchoring news shows; each of these workspaces demands the use of make-up and hair-colour. Cosmetics have become an indispensible part of our lives. The chemicals in them have a harsh impact; they urgently need to be balanced with natural products. A proper balance of both chemical and natural products is a must to maintain youthful skin and glossy hair.

Apart from balancing and taking good care of the skin, one needs to have the right attitude; one needs a beautiful mind to look beautiful. You may have perfect features but if you don't have other attributes like compassion, a sense of humour, humility, intelligence, a good sense of hygiene – in short, if you aren't groomed – these deficits will lessen the impact of physical beautiful. Beauty is a loaded term, with multiple facets, and this needs to be understood. Prettiness cannot merely be found in jars and bottles of cream.

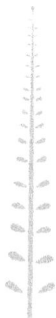

❧

I was born into a simple family where we were taught to love all that we had. My parents thought the world of me, but I was not content, simply because I was dark. I would always receive patronising, apologetic compliments: 'She's dark, but she has good features' or 'She's dark, but still, she is quite beautiful.' What I wanted was a simple statement, without a 'but'. She is beautiful. Period.

Since I belonged to a conservative family, going to beauty parlours and using chemicals was a complete no. In hindsight, I am glad. Bleaching has always been viewed as a quick-fix solution for fair skin. However, try bleaching a simple cloth piece umpteen times; see how the quality of the cloth gets affected. If this is the fate of cotton, imagine what could happen to one's delicate skin!

When I grew up, I stared delving into the riches of Ayurveda to find herbs that could lighten my complexion. I rubbed

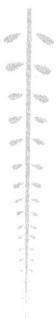

the whites of egg on my skin; this granted it smoothness, removed all facial hair, even kept my hands and legs free of hair. (Indeed, one could even use egg whites on little girls!)

I applied turmeric and lentils. My skin glowed, my face had lustre and polish, people turned to glance at me. But my quest for fair skin met with only limited success, and I remained dejected.

With time, I learnt the need to love myself. I also learnt that I owed my skin health and care, not fairness.

My experiments with Ayurveda led me to discover and create cosmetics at home, from natural ingredients, to maintain my own skin and hair. While I saw that creams and lotions were in vogue, I wanted to experiment with the extracts of herbs, fruits and flowers, and fashion something that my grandmother would approve of! I combined turmeric, green gram, sandalwood and almond, and named my little box 'Skin Toner'. I applied it religiously, and people started noticing a significant improvement in the quality of my skin. Even after a 10-hour workday, my face would still stay fresh sans makeup.

One of my friends happened to be getting married at that point. Her concern was that her skin was acne-ridden, had blemishes and an uneven colour tone. She asked me if my skin toner could help her. Initially I was reluctant, for I had only really tried this pack on myself. But finally, I relented. A few weeks of using the skin toner regularly, and lo and behold! My friend was transformed; her skin was spotless and it shone with beauty.

I started offering the skin toner to other friends and relatives, urging them to embrace a product that was wholly natural. Hesitantly, they did, and as their skins started radiating beauty, they became converts to my cause.

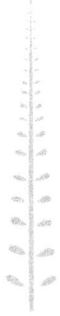

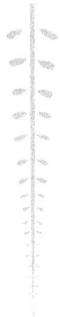

One day, while travelling by train, someone offered me my own skin toner, and said, 'Use it, it's good for the skin!' That's when I realised the benefits of my work.

Since then, there has been no looking back...

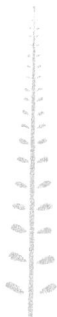

This book is an attempt at validating each and every experience of mine – as the founder of Nirmal Herbal – in using the freshest of natural ingredients to develop astringents, bleachers, scrubs and cleansers for the skin and hair. It's been 21 long years in the space, and today I can proudly say that in the midst of a massive cosmetic industry, we have established natural cures as the way forward.

To take care of your body naturally, I am here to guide you. I have borrowed the simplest of ingredients from our very own garden, kitchen, or grocer's shop, to create pastes and scrubs.

These are secrets, gathered over years of research. Today, I share them with you.

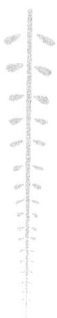

TABLE OF MEASURES

1 cup	=	200 ml
1 tbsp	=	15 ml/3 tsp
1 tsp	=	5 ml
A pinch	=	⅛ tsp
A dash	=	2 drops

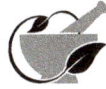

Food for Thought

Beauty is skin deep – this is a saying I often return to, and over a period of time I have reinterpreted it. I believe that anything applied on our body is absorbed by the skin. Which is why, one needs to be wary of chemicals. If we refuse to consume chemicals for breakfast or lunch, why do we impose chemicals on our bodies?

The food we eat vitalises our system, offers it minerals, vitamins and nutrients. If we dip into these food products for external application, their capacity to heal does not diminish. Nature's gifts – fruits, dry fruits, herbs, vegetables, flowers – are rich in properties that can only enhance the skin and hair. So why not fashion your cosmetics from the bounties of nature to ensure that your body is only exposed to products that are 100 per cent natural?

In doing so though, one needs to understand the term 'natural'. How natural is natural really? With the whole globe going green, with 'natural remedies' becoming buzz words in the beauty and cosmetic industry, with 'herbal from a bottle' turning into a favourite term, are we in fact leading sustainable lives? Are the products crowding the market space, claiming to have unprocessed extracts, or derivations from various organic sources, natural?

Well, the sad truth is, no. If you cut a vegetable like cucumber, it turns stale in 2 or 3 hours. How then can a cucumber last for weeks on end? The fact is, any product with a shelf life of over 3 months needs preservation; these preservatives can only be derived using chemical processes.

Which is why, I say, use the cucumber neat. Grind it daily. It requires some amount of work. But then, your body and hair glow with such care. When used naturally, the potency of every fruit, vegetable and flower doubles, and the benefits are for all to see

Each time, therefore, this book refers to 100 per cent natural products, it's fashioning them by blending fruits, vegetables, dry fruits, herbs in their freshest forms for application on the skin and hair. No preservatives are endorsed.

✻

2

Food is an integral part of our wellbeing and existence. The natural processes in our body are so rhythmic, so synchronised, that every food element is broken down and only the required portions are taken into the body. For the body to work well, only the freshest of fruits and vegetables must be consumed.

Unfortunately, in the modern world, we are bombarded with advertisements to buy and consume 'processed foods', rather than local fresh vegetables. We are offered quick-fix, 2-minute microwavable recipes; we are rarely encouraged to cook ourselves. With a growth spurt in the new processed foods industry, cheap, high calorie, nutrient poor items have become a part of everyday diet. Such food products hurt every member of society, right from children to senior citizens, across every corner of our world. Poor default food choices create problematic health conditions like obesity, diabetes, high cholesterol, and high pressure; these are all lifestyle driven diseases.

This book is a firm believer in organic food. Fresh vegetables and fruits grant the skin and hair splendour.

⚘

How can food make you look good internally? Let us go back to The Doctrine of Signatures – ancient philosophical wisdom shared by herbalists since the 15th century. It states that food that resembles various parts of the body can be used to treat ailments of that part of the body. A theological justification was made for this viewpoint: 'It was reasoned that the Almighty must have set his sign upon the various means of curing disease which he provided.'[1]

In a similar doctrine from India, the sage Agasthiar is supposed to have had the capacity to converse with plants, and learn from them the ailments and diseases they could treat, prevent and even cure.

'God's pharmacy', conceptualised by The Doctrine of Signatures, lists some food items that enhance one's inner health beauty. It says, the healing and nourishing properties of any fruit or vegetable would be reflected in, and ultimately revealed by, that fruit or vegetable's outer physical shape, form, or 'signature' in relation to the human body.

Accordingly, kidney beans actually heal and help regularise kidney function. Observe them; they are shaped exactly like the human kidneys.

A walnut looks like a little brain, a left and right hemisphere, upper cerebrums and lower cerebellums. Even the wrinkles or folds on the nut are just like the neo-cortex. We now know walnuts help develop brain function.

---

1   Andrew Dickson White, *A History of the Warfare of Science with Theology in Christendom*, Vol 2 (New York: D Appleton and Company, 1896), p 38.

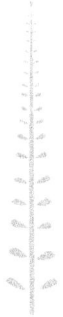

The cross section of a carrot – the pupil, iris and radiating lines – looks just like the human eye. And science now shows carrots greatly enhance blood flow to the eyes and aid in their general functioning.

Celery looks just like bones. Interestingly, celery specifically targets bone strength. Bones hold 23 per cent sodium and celery holds 23 per cent sodium too. If you don't have enough sodium in your diet, the body extracts it from the bones, thus making them weak. Foods like celery replenish the skeletal needs of the body.

Avocadoes aid the health and functioning of the womb and cervix of females. Watch them; they look just like these organs. Avocadoes help balance hormones, shed unwanted birth weight, and deter cervical cancers. Interestingly, it takes exactly 9 months for an avocado to grow from blossom to ripened fruit.

4

Figs are full of seeds and hang in twos when they grow. Predictably, they increase the mobility of male sperm, increase their number and potency; they help overcome male sterility.

Slice a mushroom in half and it resembles the human ear. Mushrooms have been found to improve hearing; indeed, they are one of the few food items to contain vitamin D. This particular vitamin helps develop healthy bones, even the tiny ones in the ear that transmit sound to the brain.

Now, let's consider grapes, which grow in clusters on vines. Our lungs are made up of branches of airways that finish up with tiny bunches of tissue called alveoli. These structures allow oxygen to pass from the lungs to the blood stream. Do you spot a similarity between grapes and our lungs? A diet high in fresh fruit, such as grapes, has been shown to reduce the risk of lung cancer and emphysema. Grape seeds also contain a chemical called proanthocyanidin,

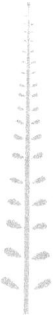

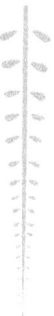

which appears to reduce the severity of asthma triggered by allergy.

Ginger, commonly sold in supermarkets, often looks just like the stomach. So it's interesting that one of its biggest benefits is aiding digestion. The Chinese have been using ginger for over 2,000 years to calm the stomach and cure nausea; ginger is also a popular remedy for motion sickness.

Sweet potatoes look like the pancreas and actually balance the glycemic index of diabetics.

Finally, observe the magnificent olive. Isn't it shaped like the female ovary? Believe it or not, olives assist with the health and functioning of the ovaries.

Today, we have several food institutions that have re-discovered the principles of The Doctrine of Signatures, and promote a lifestyle that's healthy and balanced.

❧

5

Some people are allergic to specific natural ingredients. If you sense you are allergic, we recommend a patch test to avoid adverse reactions.

I also recommend a skin analysis. Get your skin tested, evaluate your skin type, then dip into beauty products. This is because the products you use, and the way you use them would depend on the results of a skin analysis. For instance, almond – which has bleaching properties – could simply be ground, without soaking, when used on dry skin. But in the case of those with oily skin, almonds can only be ground and used after soaking them overnight.

Most of all, I believe that anything done with a touch of love works. If I massage someone who has a headache with tenderness, I bring relief. If I dab a face pack with a mother's touch on an anxious teenager, the pack is bound to work wonders.

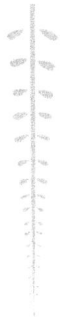

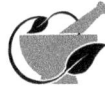

General Notes
regarding natural recipes

- All packs should be freshly prepared and used, for maximum benefit, unless otherwise stated. Storage can interfere with the efficiency of the product.

- If required, each pack could be stored in a refrigerator for a day.

- While we have provided measures for each listed ingredient, we're not rigid. A major advantage with regard to herbal products is that the ingredients, even when not in exact proportion, still offer excellent benefits.

- All leaves, herbs, vegetables, used directly or ground, should be washed well prior.

- If 2 sets of ingredients are to be ground, ensure that separate blending machines are used. Else, wash the vessels and grinders well!

- Those with sensitive skin should do a patch test on their neck to check suitability before applying the pack.

- When mixing aromatic oils, use a glass bowl or container. Aromatic oils should never be used neat, but should be added to oils, juices or water.

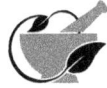

The Wonders of
Common Kitchen Ingredients

Let's remember Hippocrates who said: Let food be thy medicine.

Natural foods are treasures filled with goodness, and are a must for sound health. Regular intake of fresh fruits and vegetables ensures great skin and hair.

Our ancestors used food as cosmetics. And I, personally, strongly believe that what is good for your stomach is good for your skin. Indeed, the best part of going natural is that you're in nature's good hands; there is no likelihood that you will regret your decision!

Here are some easy-to-make home remedies, as simple as daily cooking. Only remember to prepare fresh packs and wait patiently for the results to show.

Happy cooking!

A

Almond

Almonds are one of the greatest beauty aids, whether used as dried powder, soaked or ground.

The almond – blessed with proteins, vitamins B and E, Omega-3 fatty acids and nutrients – nourishes the skin, brightens it and removes traces of pigmentation. Rich in antioxidants, it protects the skin from the sun's harmful rays and slows the ageing process. The abundance of protein found in it acts as a building block for skin, and the calcium helps the body absorb nutrients.

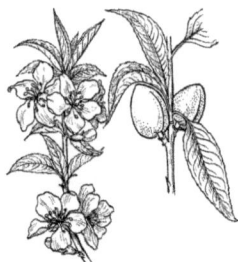

Almonds can be used for those with oily skin, in which case, they need to be soaked, peeled and ground. For those with dry skin, they can be ground without soaking.

Aloe Vera

Aloe vera is a rare plant indeed! It contains multiple vitamins, including A, C, B1, B2, B3, B6 and E! Aloe vera is also one of the few plants that contains vitamin B12. Almost 20 minerals are found in it, including calcium, copper, magnesium, potassium and zinc.

Aloe vera, as a result, is enormously popular in the cosmetic trade. It soothes the skin, and prevents itchiness. Since it contains over 99 per cent water, aloe vera hydrates, moisturises, nourishes

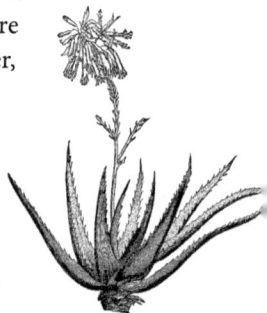

and revitalises the skin. It increases its elasticity, softens it, and allows the skin to soak in oxygen!

Aloe vera juice, according to ancient Ayurveda, fights Pitta-related ailments. In the case of rosacea, it protects the outer layers of the skin, and reduces inflammation.

While its skin benefits are well known, aloe vera also nourishes the hair. Extract the pulp from an aloe plant to treat your hair with an amazing conditioner!

Amla (Indian Gooseberry)

Amla, as a fruit, is known for its innumerable health benefits, both internal and external. Indeed, according to Ayurveda, regular use of amla balances all 3 doshas; its cooling properties stabilise Vata and Pitta, while its drying properties balance Kapha.

Highly rich in vitamin C – a glass of amla juice contains 20 times more vitamin C than a glass of fresh orange juice – amla is known to be one of nature's best immunity builders. Besides this, amla is also known to be rich in minerals like iron, phosphorus and calcium. It is fortified with antioxidants, and a regular glass of amla juice retards the ageing process.

Given the many treasures this magic berry holds, it is used to address multiple ailments, from diabetes to asthma. It is also used extensively to cure hair problems. Amla extracts make excellent oils and shampoos to battle dandruff; amla tonics also darken hair and check hair fall.

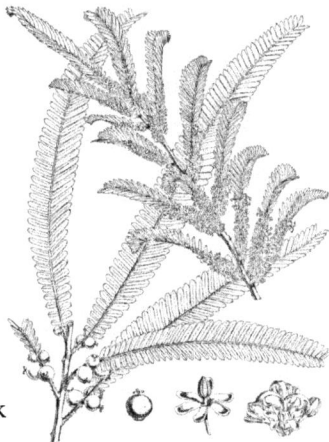

11

Apple

The clichéd proverb – an apple a day keeps the doctor away – isn't wholly myth. And if apples are consumed and also applied externally, their impact doubles!

Apples are extremely beneficial with regard to skin health. Rich in vitamins A, B and C, they feed the skin! Apples also exfoliate, and have excellent antioxidant properties. These antioxidant compounds, called phenols, provide UV protection, making your skin resistant to damage from the sun. Besides, the apple's antioxidant compounds prevent cell and tissue damage.

Apples contain abundant amounts of elastin and collagen that help keep the skin young. Equally, this miracle fruit makes for a good face pack for those with open pores on their skin. Lastly, apples make the skin glow!

In this regard, it is also important to mention apple cider vinegar, and its properties. Apple cider vinegar is a well-known astringent for acne-prone skin, with definite antifungal and antibacterial properties. Its alpha-hydroxy acids remove dead skin. Apart from relieving the skin of excess oils, it helps balance pH levels and normalise sebum production.

Apricot

Apricots hold vitamins A and C, calcium, potassium, phosphorus, iron and fatty acids.

The fatty acids make apricots excellent moisturisers. The oil derived from the common apricot is mild, gentle, and non-greasy, gets absorbed almost

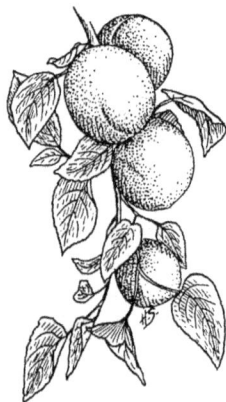

immediately by the skin, and hydrates it. Besides, the oil contains gamma linoleic acid that firms and tones the body. Vitamins A and E in the meantime slow down physical signs of ageing.

Given its hydrating properties, the oil derived from the apricot is used to condition hair, granting it extra softness.

Apricots are often used in exfoliating scrubs, for their kernels sough off dead skin cells, unclog pores, and encourage new cells to grow.

Apricots finally have anti-inflammatory properties that soothe those suffering from eczema and dermatitis.

Avocado

Avocadoes are storehouses of vitamins A, D and E, as also H.

13

These nutrients promise to keep the skin moisturised, and soften it. Simply running the pulp of a mashed avocado across the face, and washing this off with lukewarm water after 15 minutes, helps hydrate dry skin. Moreover, the vitamin E in avocado fights environmental damage.

Similarly, avocado oil rejuvenates and moisturises the scalp, and revitalises dry, lifeless hair.

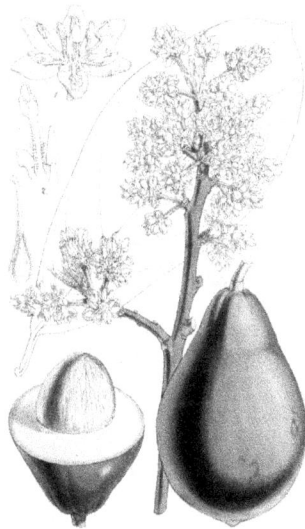

B

Banana

Bananas are rich in iron, potass
vitamins A, B, B6 and B12, as also mang
and antioxidants. Given their compo
bananas act against ageing, and maintain the
elasticity of the skin.

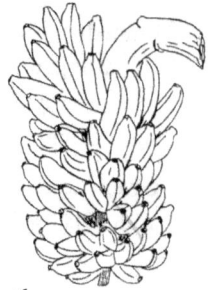

Besides, bananas have a high degree of water content; as a result they hydrate the skin and prevent it from drying and chapping. The peels of a banana contain lutein, a powerful antioxidant, which helps treat dry, itchy skin. Lastly, the generous doses of vitamin C in the fruit grant the skin a glow.

Bananas also address hair issues. A banana hair mask helps increase the hair's moisture content, reduces a dry scalp's itchiness, and settles frizz.

Beetroot

Beetroot is fortified with vitamins A, C and K, minerals, and silica. Besides, it contains a pigment, which is known as betalain, which not only grants the vegetable its rich colour, but also acts as a powerful fungicidal, antioxidant, and anti-inflammatory agent.

Not surprisingly, beetroot brings out the best in one's skin and hair. In fact, regular consumption of beetroot juice, combined with carrots and cucumbers, helps add a glow to the skin.

Since beetroot is a natural dye, mixing it with henna grants one's hair an auburn glow. One of beet juice's best kept secrets is that it helps clear stubborn dandruff.

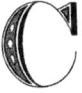

C

Carrot

Rich in vitamin A, carrots help maintain healthy skin and prevent acne.

One of the best ways of making skin luminous is by pampering it with antioxidant agents. Carrots, with high levels of antioxidants, help balance the pH factor, prevent free radical damage, and make the skin joyful! Indeed, carrots contain a special antioxidant, carotenoid, which keep the face glowing.

Carrot juice is an excellent lightening agent. Apply carrot juice on blemishes and leave it overnight. Over a period of time, you will notice that the scars and blemishes have faded.

15

The potassium content of carrot removes traces of skin pigmentation and promotes excellent complexion. Simply applying carrot juice on one's skin helps in skin brightening too!

Clove

Cloves hold calcium, iron and magnesium.

They are perhaps best known for their antiseptic and germicidal properties. As a result, clove based products are often recommended as cures for fungal infections.

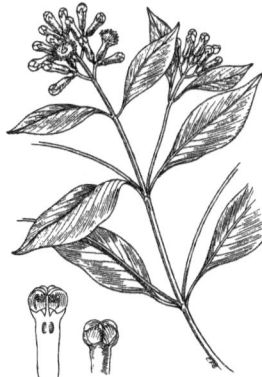

Equally, cloves are recommended to fight acne. Cloves are fortified with eugenol, which is known as an antibacterial compound. Cloves therefore rid the skin of cystic acne, kill infection, and reduce swelling. Merely dabbing cystic zits with a pinch of clove powder in water can work wonders. However do be careful, since cloves can irritate sensitive skin.

Coconut

Coconut is one of my own favourite beauty foods, as every part of it – from the water, to the milk, the oil, and the pulp – can be used to treat skin and hair. Wow! That makes it nature's all-purpose gift!

Coconut, which holds vitamin E, helps scars and other skin discolorations fade. As for its water, it has the highest concentration of electrolytes among all natural food items, and therefore hydrates!

16

Whether ingested or applied to the skin, coconut milk has a range of properties! It contains within it the goodness of vitamins B1, B3, B5, B6, C and E, as well as sodium, iron, calcium, magnesium and phosphorus. It hydrates the skin and keeps it soft and smooth. Its fat content locks in moisture. And its copper and vitamin C contents keep skin supple! Further, it is a great nourishing ingredient for hair, keeping it soft; it also helps darken it.

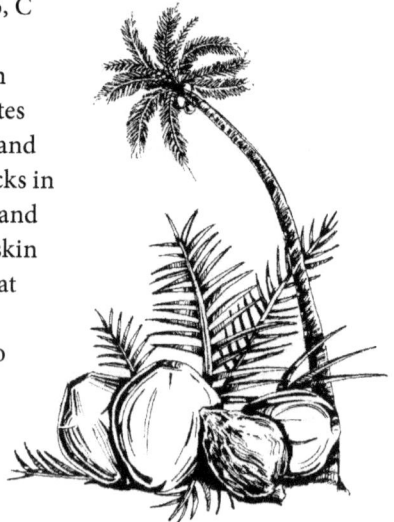

Cucumber

Cucumbers are rich in vitamin C, silicon, sulphur and antioxidants.

These are all ingredients that benefit the skin and hair. While vitamin C helps soothe skin irritations and reduce swelling, a cucumber's high silicon content makes hair healthy. Cucumbers work as super astringents, cooling and brightening agents for skin.

From dark circles to puffy eyes, cucumbers address a number of beauty issues. The antioxidants in cucumber are gentle enough to nourish the skin around the eyes, while the ascorbic acid in the vegetable decreases water retention and therefore puffiness. For good skin, applying cucumber juice daily either on its own or mixed with other ingredients is a must, for it acts as a wonderful natural toner.

Curry Leaf

Curry leaves are storehouses of vitamins A and C, phosphorus, iron and calcium.

Curry leaves are nature's gift to the hair. They are known to prevent premature greying, nourish hair follicles and the root, fight dandruff and stimulate hair growth. The innocuous curry leaf is the ideal cure for almost all hair problems!

Consuming curry leaves also helps control premature greying.

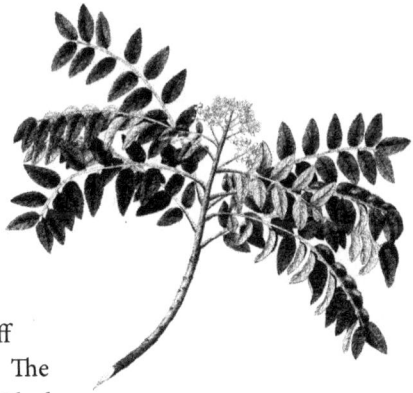

D

Drumstick Leaf

As in the case of the coconut, almost every part of the tree growing drumsticks is valuable, from the flower and seeds, to the leaves, roots and even the gum!

Drumstick leaves are fortified with vitamins A, C and E. They hold twice more calcium than milk, and 3 times more iron than spinach. If consumed orally, by opting for a soup made of drumstick leaves, the body gets huge amounts of calcium.

Drumstick leaves are known for their antibacterial properties. Since they are purifying agents, they help cleanse the skin. Moreover, they possess anti-ageing properties, clearing skin cells of free radicals and making the face young and fresh.

The leaves are good for the hair too, because they hold high levels of iron and calcium, and show traces of B-complex.

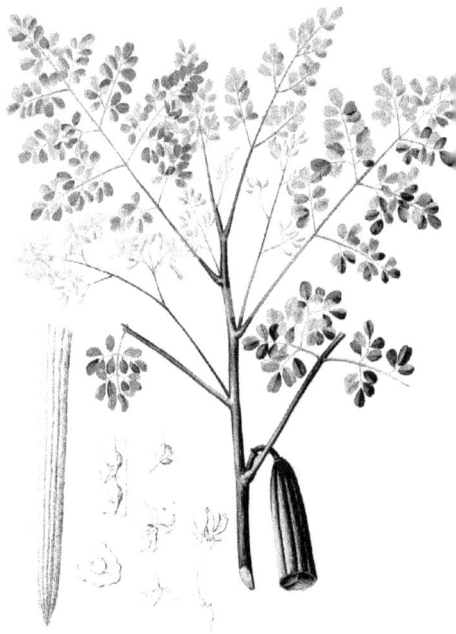

E

Egg

Rich in vitamins A ,B, D and E along with protein and zinc, eggs are great for the skin and hair.

The whites are known to reduce oiliness, and are useful for those with acne-prone skin. The yolk is valuable for those with dry skin. The fat in the egg helps moisturise and soften skin.

Besides, eggs are great for the hair. You may well ask why. It's because eggs have huge reserves of protein. Our hair is composed of 70 per cent keratin protein, and the application of eggs fortifies each strand by feeding it. Hair therefore is granted strength and lustre!

19

F

Fenugreek (Methi)

Fenugreek seeds contain vitamin C, protein, niacin, potassium, calcium and carotene.

Fenugreek is a great hair saver, helps treat follicular problems and strengthens hair. Since it holds proteins and nicotinic acid, apart from lecithin – a natural emollient – it addresses problems associated with dry, damaged and dandruff-prone hair.

G

Gelatin

Gelatin is fortified with protein especially keratin. Indeed, every tablespoon of gelatin holds 6 grams of protein.

Gelatin is also largely composed of the amino acids, glycine and proline. These rarely get consumed since the acids are found in the bones and fibrous tissues of animals. However, including them in your diet is important since they help build healthy skin, hair and nails.

Not surprisingly, gelatin is especially useful if you wish to strengthen your nails.

Green Gram Lentil

Green gram lentils are loaded with vitamins B and C, proteins, calcium, magnesium, and fibre.

Green gram is an excellent substitute to body soap, since it scrubs off dirt. Furthermore, it removes surplus oil from the back, and thus checks the spread of acne. Finally, since it is rich in protein, it helps the skin build new, healthy cells, and grants the body sheen.

Green gram is equally effective if dealing with dandruff. Green gram powder may be used instead of a shampoo, since it can remove dirt, soothe, hydrate, and prevent flaking.

H

Hibiscus

This scarlet flower is known for its cooling properties. Rich in vitamin C, it also holds a range of organic acids, including citric, malic and tartaric acids. It also contains allo-hydroxycitric acid lactone, or hibiscus acid, which is unique to the flower.

The hibiscus is best known to nurture hair. The commonly found flower has been used for centuries to treat various hair disorders. It is known to encourage hair growth by stimulating circulation, prevent premature greying and split ends, and battle dandruff.

Moreover, its rich red hue acts as great hair colour, especially when combined with henna. The hibiscus grants one smooth and glossy tresses. The leaves could be ground and used as a conditioner for hair.

21

Holy Basil (Tulsi)

Holy basil is known as the queen of herbs, as the most sacred of all the aromatic plants in India. Holy basil contains the goodness of vitamins A, C, E, K, potassium, manganese, iron, copper, and antioxidants such as eugenol.

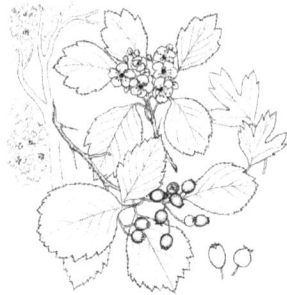

Holy basil can be eaten directly. Consuming a handful of these leaves boiled with half a teaspoon of honey helps relieve stress, purify the blood and cleanse the skin.

Holy basil is endowed with antiseptic, antifungal, and antibacterial qualities. This, along with the fact that it purifies the blood of toxins, makes it an excellent fighter of not only pimples but also conditions like ringworm and eczema.

Holy basil, further, is known to have extraordinarily powerful antioxidant properties that can protect the body from premature ageing.

It is also known to shield the skin from the sun. The herb contains the flavonoids, orientin and vicenin, plant pigments that protect skin cells from radiation damage. Holy basil, when applied on sunburnt skin, is a soothing agent.

Honey

Honey contains both fructose and glucose, natural sweeteners that nourish. Besides it is full of nutrients like vitamin B6, copper, iron, manganese, calcium, sodium and potassium.

Honey is nature's natural anti-ageing gel. Centuries ago, Cleopatra, the Egyptian queen, used to take luxurious baths in milk and honey to remain youthful in appearance. Even today, grandmothers recommend face packs made with this gel. The reason is that honey can make the skin elastic, smoothen out fine lines and reduce the appearance of wrinkles.

Besides, honey is a natural humectant, attracts and retains moisture from the air, and keeps the skin naturally hydrated. Because the moisture gets sealed in, the skin feels soft and supple.

Honey has antioxidant, antimicrobial, antifungal and antibacterial properties. As a result, it draws out impurities from the skin, targets breakouts, reduces redness and calms inflammation.

Honey is an excellent exfoliator, even for sensitive or problem skin; it is mild enough to use daily, unlike several chemical exfoliators that irritate with the passage of time.

Finally, honey not only protects the skin from the sun, but also soothes if one gets sunburnt. Dab a drop of honey on sun-damaged skin, and watch it heal!

I

Indian Pennywort (Brahmi)

Indian pennywort contains vitamins B1, B2, B3 and B6, as well as the minerals calcium, magnesium, sodium, manganese and zinc.

Indian pennywort is known as the longevity herb, because it helps rebuild tissue, rejuvenate skin, and slow the ageing process.

23

Besides, Indian pennywort, with its excellent antifungal and antibacterial properties, can be used to treat eczema, psoriasis, and other skin conditions.

Indian pennywort is a miracle herb for the hair, granting strength to the roots, stimulating growth, promoting follicular nourishment, and preventing dandruff. An Indian pennywort hair oil massage will leave you with shiny, healthy hair.

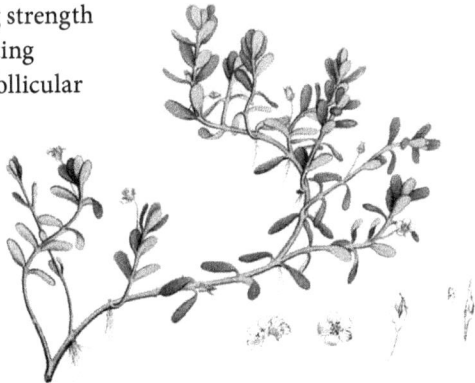

J

Jasmine

Jasmine flowers are not just sweet smelling, but are also packed with vitamin C.

In aromatherapy, jasmine is used to calm emotions, and produce feelings of self-confidence, happiness and hope. Jasmine is used in hair oils both for its scent as also because it nourishes.

K

Khus Khus (Poppy Seeds)

Khus khus is fortified with omega-3 fatty acids, vitamin E, and various minerals including manganese, zinc, copper and magnesium.

It not only acts as an ideal aromatic coolant to beat the summer heat, but also has anti-inflammatory and antiseptic properties.

Besides, khus khus, when ground into a paste with milk, is known to act as an excellent moisturiser that refreshes and renews skin cells. The natural oils in it keep skin supple, while the linolec acid treats eczema, burning sensations and itching.

Khus khus is also effective if attempting to address dark patches under the eyes.

Finally, since khus khus is an opium based seed, it is known to help one relax!

Please note though: It is advisable to do a patch test as some people are allergic to khus khus.

L

Lavender

Lavender is rich in vitamins A and C, calcium and iron.

Its oil is especially known for its antiseptic and antifungal properties, which help to reduce skin scarring and accelerate healing. Just dabbing lavender oil with a cotton pod on acne can reduce inflammation. Equally, lavender oil helps treat eczema, by relieving itching and soreness.

Lavender has long been used for aromatherapy, and is known to reduce tension. Indeed, several books speak of women in the Victorian era keeping lavender sachets in their pockets to fight stress. Since contentment and beauty are closely linked, lavender is known to bring a youthful glow to the skin.

Given its reputation for stemming tension, lavender is used for manicures and pedicures, to treat harassed hands and feet. Equally, it is used to address hair problems; by reducing anxiety and worry – the root cause of several hair issues – it ensures that our tresses remain healthy and full of bounce!

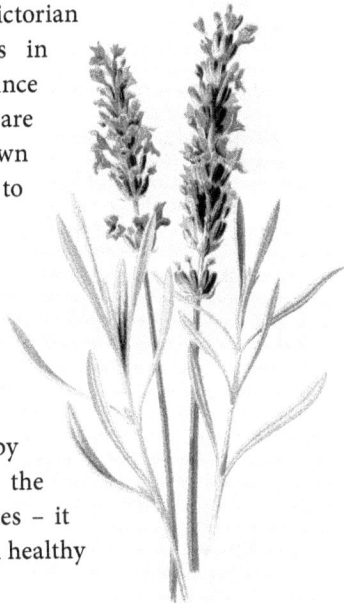

Lime

Do not mistake limes for lemons! Look closely and you can spot the difference. Lemons are light yellow and sport thick, rough skins, while limes are greenish-yellow and have fine skins.

Lime is full of vitamin C, as also potassium and phosphorus. Due to its antiseptic and antibacterial properties, as also its sweet fragrance, lime extracts are used in several hair and skin products.

Lime is excellent for treating dry or rough skin and moisturising. In case of oily skin, lime can act as an astringent or skin tonic.

It also helps improve skin tone. The mild bleaching agents in it help get rid of pigmentation, spots and blemishes. Indeed, lime extracts can even be used to lighten underarms and knees.

26

Even the peel of lime is of value, since if ground and applied on pimples, it can help get rid of them.

In spite of its good properties, lime juice should never be used directly. It however could be mixed with some medium like milk, buttermilk or water and used on the skin.

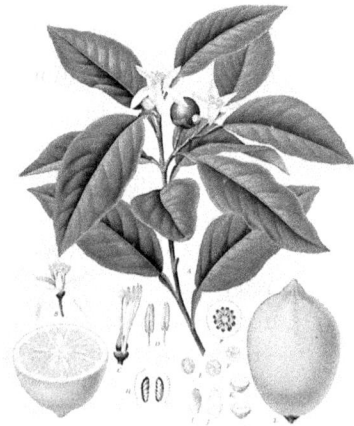

M

Margosa (Neem)

In the ancient Vedas, the margosa tree is referred to as Sarva Roga Nirvarini – one that can cure every illness and ailment. As a result, margosa has been used for centuries to fight health disorders. Every part of the tree, be it the branches and leaves or the roots and flowers, is beneficial.

Margosa contains the azadirachtin compound which gives it antibacterial, antifungal and antiparasitic properties. Its leaves hold within them vitamin C, proteins, calcium, phosphorus, carotene, as also several fatty acids.

Margosa has immune system stimulating compounds; consequently, with its aid, the skin fights pathogens and remains without flaws. The paste of margosa leaves cures many diseases that affect the skin, including chicken pox, small pox, and measles. It also fights fungal infections such as ringworm.

Margosa helps relieve dry, itchy skin, and addresses conditions like eczema and psoriasis; the vitamin E and fatty acids in it penetrate the skin and prevents a loss of moisture.

When applied on acne-prone skin, margosa reduces redness and inflammation and tightens pores; its fatty acids help treat acne scarring; its astringent qualities cure sore pimples.

Weekly application of margosa oil ensures that the scalp and hair remain healthy. It acts as a natural cure for dandruff, rejuvenates a dry scalp, and prevents itchiness. It also promotes hair growth and strengthens each strand; as a result it prevents breakage, thinning and hair loss. Margosa oil has been used for centuries to battle hair lice too!

27

Marigold

Marigolds are fortified with vitamins A, B1 and D.

These flowers address dry, sensitive, damaged skin. Equally, marigolds have anti-inflammatory and antiseptic qualities. Boiled and mashed marigolds have long been used to heal cuts, blemishes, acne and rashes, as well as battle dermatitis and eczema.

Marigolds are also known for their antioxidant properties, and for protecting the skin from free radicals. They have been used to fight ageing and wrinkles, and to revitalise sagging skin.

Because of their natural astringent and antibacterial properties, marigolds are also used to revive brittle hair and soothe the scalp.

Milk

Milk, fortified with vitamins A, D and E, is often a component in several skin and hair packs.

Milk, first and foremost, has moisturising properties. The fats and proteins in it hydrate the body. It's for this reason that the queens of yore used to have milk baths! Their skins would glow. Besides, the moisturising properties of milk also address itching caused by eczema.

Given its qualities, milk also occasionally figures as an ingredient in natural hair washes. It helps treat dry, lifeless, damaged locks. Again, the queens of ancient India were known to dip their tresses in pools of milk to rejuvenate them.

The fat in milk helps treat inflammation; it eases the redness caused by sunburn and sun-damage.

Curd, derived from milk, possesses several of its healing properties. Additionally, the probiotics in it soothe irritated skin, the high zinc content fights acne and closes pores, and the lactic acid combats ageing!

Mint

Mint leaves are rich in vitamins A, C, D and E as also minerals like calcium, phosphorus, and iron, and salicylic acid.

Mint is an active ingredient in cleansers, moisturisers, shampoos, conditioners, and of course, lip balms. This is because it is known to soften and calm the skin.

Equally, mint is known for its anti-inflammatory properties. Mint can be applied to soothe mosquito bites; it can also be used to combat acne. The salicylic acid in mint addresses stubborn zits and blackheads, loosens up dead skin cells, and prevents the pores from getting clogged. The vitamin A in the meantime controls oiliness and refreshes!

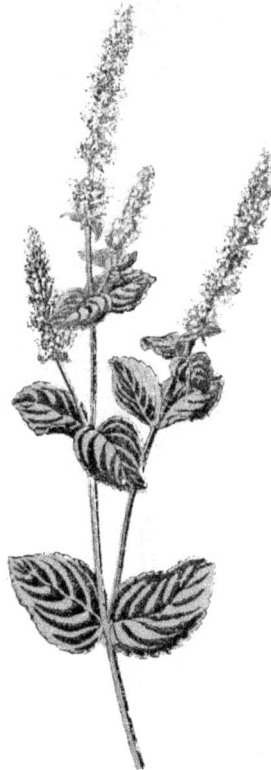

29

N

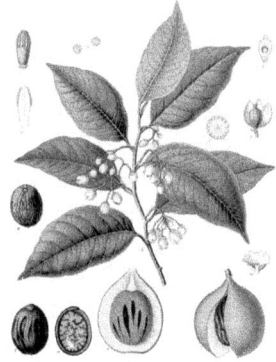

Nutmeg

Nutmegs are a storehouse of vitamins A and C, potassium, copper and manganese.

Nutmegs have been used in various Ayurvedic potions since ancient times to treat skin ailments. Minute quantities are sufficient to derive all the benefits.

Nutmegs, with their antiseptic properties, are best known as acne fighters. They help one attain smooth, flawless skin. A scrub of nutmeg powder and a little rice powder can help remove blackheads, excess oil and dead skin cells. Equally, nutmeg addresses scarring. A simple paste of nutmeg powder and oats, when applied regularly to spots and scars, leaves you with smooth, glowing skin!

Nutmegs may be a little strong for those with sensitive skin, and therefore should be used with care.

30

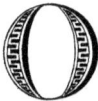

Oat

Rich in vitamin E, zinc magnesium, phosphorus, potassium, selenium and fibre, oats speak to all skin types – be it oily, or dry, or acne ridden. While a teenager could use oatmeal as a mild cleanser to ease sebum secretion, someone with ageing skin would benefit from an oatmeal scrub! Oats are natural cleansers, no matter the skin type, and can quite easily replace cosmetic face scrubs.

Oatmeal is an excellent natural remedy for treating acne. If applied on the affected area for 10 minutes, oatmeal absorbs excess oil and bacteria, exfoliates, and battles acne.

In case of dull, flaky skin, the polisaccharides in oats (which become gelatinous in water) form a protective, nourishing, hydrating film on the skin. Not surprisingly, oats can also address itchy skin and offer immediate relief. A softening pack of oatmeal could be used by those suffering from eczema or psoriasis to ease the desire to scratch.

Oats are known as skin lighteners too; they fight acne scars and spots, and even out freckled areas. Besides, the proteins in oatmeal act as barriers and protect the skin from the harsh rays of the sun.

Oatmeal also eases wrinkles.

Orange

Oranges are fortified with vitamin C, and also have reserves of vitamin A, copper and iron.

Oranges soothe the face on summer days. They detoxify the skin, and make it luminous. Fresh orange juice grants the skin vitamin C. When mixed with honey, and applied to the face and neck, it feeds dull and dehydrated facial skin.

Oranges also combat acne; their peels are said to cure blemishes, open pores and blackheads. The citric acid in the fruit is an astringent that dries away zits! Is your skin pimple-prone? Grind an orange peel and apply it on your pimples regularly.

Furthermore, being rich in antioxidants, oranges help firm and tone the skin, and fight wrinkles.

Oranges act as natural bleaches, lighten tans, and come without the corrosive side effects of chemical bleaches. As a result, they are often active ingredients in facial lotions and cleansers.

P

Papaya

Loaded with vitamins A, C and E, potassium, magnesium and fibre, papaya makes for excellent skin food.

It also contains papain, a natural skin enzyme that activates skin renewal and cell turnover. As a result, papaya is often an active ingredient in masks that promise exfoliation. Mashed papaya is also strongly recommended for treating sore and cracked heels, so dead cells are soughed off, and fresh skin can form.

Moreover, papaya helps battle blemishes. Apply papaya paste on the face for 15 minutes, and wash it off with lukewarm water. On regular application, those uncomfortable pimples will vanish!

Papaya is excellent as hair food, for it prevents balding, controls dandruff, washes off dirt, boosts shaft strength, and adds to hair volume.

Pistachio

Pistachios are endowed with vitamins A, B6 and C, magnesium, calcium and iron.

These dry fruits are best known for their anti-ageing properties. The vitamin E in pistachios fight the ageing process. The antioxidants neutralise free radicals and

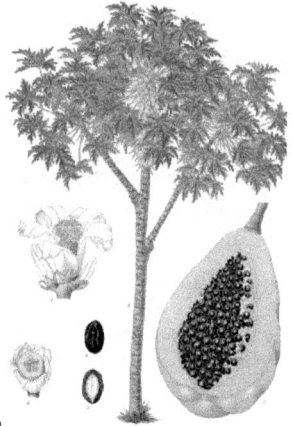

protect the skin from harmful UV rays. And the natural oils hydrate the skin and prevent it from drying.

Indeed, pistachios are excellent moisturisers, and pistachio oil is an ideal substitute for over-the-counter chemical moisturisers. This dry fruit's oil has demulcent properties. In other words, pistachio oil is enormously hydrating, and softens and smoothens the body.

Potato

The merits of the ubiquitous potato cannot be overstated. With vitamins A, C, B, phosphorus, calcium, iron, potassium, fibre and protein, this vegetable is an all-in-one exfoliant, healer, soother and brightener.

Potatoes help reduce burn scars and pigmentation. They work as skin lighteners and brighteners. Simply grind peeled potatoes, apply the blend to the face, then wash it off, to get rid of spots and freckles. Keep cotton balls dipped in potato juice also reduce dark circles and under-eye puffiness.

Potatoes gently exfoliate, help stimulate cell renewal, and revitalise skin. Not surprisingly, potatoes are said to fight wrinkles.

The potassium in them, in the meantime, promotes healing. Potatoes, consequently, help treat sunburnt skin. Merely applying cold potato slices on the damaged areas cools and restores.

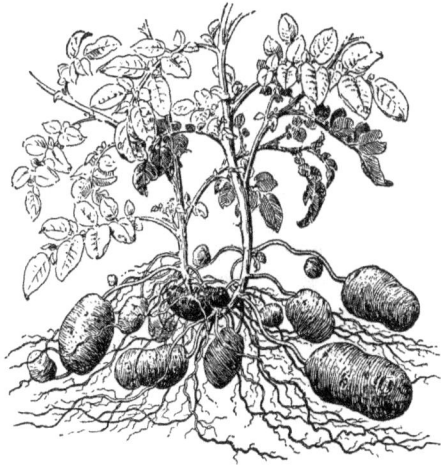

R

Red Lentil

Red lentils, also known as masoor dal, provide vitamins B6 and C, calcium, iron and potassium.

Red lentils have exfoliating properties, and can be used in body scrubs. Soak red lentils overnight, grind them, and mix them with honey (if you need moisturising) or milk. Apply this paste while in the shower, and wash off after 15 minutes with lukewarm water. The paste soughs off dead skin, revitalises the body and makes it baby soft.

Equally, red lentils grant the body a glow, and lighten scars. A paste of ground red lentils and milk is especially useful if you wish to fight a tan.

34

Finally, red lentils purify the skin, and therefore are agents that fight acne and blackheads.

Rice

Rice is rich in vitamins E, K and B6, and protein. Besides, it contains pitera, which is known to revive tired skin and lend it a glow.

Powdered rice grains are used as a body scrub since they make the skin soft. Brown rice powder is used for exfoliation and removing dead skin; it can also help treat blackheads.

Rice water has been used for centuries for beautiful skin. Simply dipping a cotton pod in rice water, and applying is across your washed face tightens pores and revitalises cells. As a result rice water is often viewed as an excellent skin toner.

The same rice water is considered to be an exceptional hair conditioner. After shampooing, all you need to do is rinse your hair with rice water, leave it on for 10 minutes, then wash it off with cold water. Your tresses will be lustrous.

Rosewater

Rose petals contain vitamins B, C, and K, besides calcium, potassium, copper and iodine. Rosewater is derived from the petals of consumable roses.

If you're making rosewater at home, wash the petals of pink consumable roses, boil them in filtered water; once the petals turn white and the water acquires a pinkish hue, filter the water, cool and refrigerate it. This is rosewater you can use.

Rosewater is perhaps best known for its cooling, soothing effects. Splash a bowl of rosewater across your face in the morning, and you will feel refreshed!

Rosewater is a great cleanser. Soak a cotton ball in rosewater and wipe your face with this. All traces of grime and dirt, even makeup, will disappear!

Rosewater also acts as a toner that tightens the pores and helps reduces fine lines and wrinkles. Its antioxidants regenerate skin tissues, while stimulating circulation. Grandmothers often recommend adding sandalwood powder to rosewater, to make a marvellous anti-ageing face mask!

Rosewater is known for its antimicrobial and antiseptic properties. It is one of nature's gentlest doctors to fight zits and heal acne wounds across all skin types. A herbal face pack comprising sandalwood powder and rosewater, when applied to the face for 15 minutes, and washed off with cold water, cures all pimple problems! Please note though: Sandalwood can also cause allergies or make the skin dry.

Thus it is advisable to do a patch test and then use the pack.

Rosewater lightens tans. Just 2 tablespoons of tomato juice mixed with an equal amount of rosewater, when applied to the face for 15 minutes, and washed off, fades tans and eases stinging sunburns.

Rosewater helps maintain the pH balance of the skin. If you have dry skin, add a dash of glycerine to rosewater and you have a natural moisturiser! If you have oily skin, add a pinch of camphor in rosewater, and the surface oiliness will reduce!

Finally, given its aroma, rosewater has a soothing effect on the nerves, relieves stress and works as an antidepressant. As we know, a cheerful disposition lends a glow to the skin.

Saffron

The stamen of the extraordinary saffron flower holds multiple beauty secrets. It is rich in vitamins A and C, folic acid, magnesium, potassium, copper and zinc.

Saffron is gifted with antibacterial qualities. It therefore treats acne, and prevents new eruptions.

Equally saffron is known for its exfoliating and skin lightening properties. It not only helps battle pimple scars, but also reduces dark circles around the eyes, harsh tans, and spots from old eruptions. Milk mixed with a few strands of saffron, when massaged across dry skin, provides a fresh rush of blood circulation, fades discolorations, and grants the face a glow.

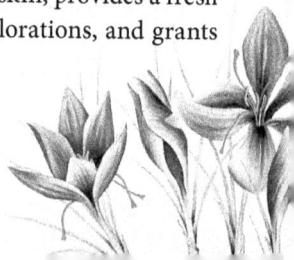

Sandalwood

The sandalwood tree's semi-parasitic nature makes it nutrient-rich, for it absorbs the minerals of its surroundings. Fortified with potassium, it is highly cooling, and has antiseptic, astringent and anti-inflammatory properties.

A paste made from sandalwood therefore helps clear the skin of acne, blackheads and skin eruptions. Mix equal quantities of sandalwood powder and turmeric powder, add a pinch of saffron and water, and get a smooth paste. Apply this on the face and neck, leave on for 5 minutes. Those stubborn pimples will die.

Sandalwood oil effectively reduces skin itching, and soothes, whether one suffers from eczema or prickly heat. Sandalwood paste mixed with rosewater is especially effective if addressing prickly heat.

Sandalwood has excellent moisturising properties. Sandalwood oil is known to hydrate dull skin.

37

Sandalwood also lightens tanned complexions, and fades acne spots. Sandalwood powder mixed with almond powder and milk, when applied to the face, instantly reduces uneven tans, blemish marks and freckles. Not only this, sandalwood has youth-granting properties.

Sandalwood however is best remembered for its strong aroma! If you suffer from body odour, simply apply sandalwood paste on your body before taking bath. It not only lessens sweating, but also grants your body a mesmerising fragrance.

It is this fragrance that the cosmetic industry dips into, for it is believed to promote sensuality and relieve tension. And as we've learnt, a stress-free mind makes for a gorgeous body!

Soap Nut

Commonly known as reetha, soap nut comes from the soap nut tree. Soap nuts are fortified with saponin, which when dissolved in water, produces mild suds. These fight odour, and have antifungal properties.

Soap nuts have been used for washing the hair since ancient times, and figure as the main ingredient in herbal shampoos. A great cleanser, soap nuts promote hair growth and keep the scalp free from dandruff. Moreover, they help battle lice!

Those with sensitive scalps find soap nuts especially useful since they are entirely natural and are hypoallergenic. Therefore, they cannot irritate the skin!

Strawberry

Strawberries are not only delicious, but also work miracles for the skin, since they are blessed with vitamin C and salicylic acids.

Strawberries are great cleansers. The salicylic acid soughs off dead skin cells and closes open pores; ellagic acid acts as an antioxidant and prevents skin damage; the vitamin C repairs tissue.

Strawberries are also toners. Besides, they perform a couple of important roles. First, they struggle against free radicals and keep the skin youthful. Second, they protect the skin from the sun's harsh and potentially harmful rays, and keep the skin healthy.

Strawberries have skin lightening properties, and battle tans, freckles and age spots. Merely applying strawberry juice across the face and washing it off in 15 minutes grants your face a sheen.

Strawberries are often found in anti-acne face washes. This is because the alpha hydroxy acids (AHAs) and salicylic acid in them stem sebum production and prevent acne outbreaks.

Finally, strawberries are great for pampering your eyes! Cut 2 slivers of the fruit and apply it to closed eyes. The puffiness and dark circles will diminish and fade in just 20 minutes!

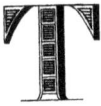

T

Tea Tree Oil

Aboriginal tribes have known of the magical properties of tea tree oil for centuries; the miracle essential oil is now available worldwide. Derived from the tea tree, a native of Australia, this oil contains cineole and terpinen, which have antibacterial and anti-inflammatory properties.

As a result, tea tree oil is especially useful while treating acne. A dash of tea tree oil, when applied to a zit, provides immediate relief! It not only acts as a germicide, but also reduces sebum secretion and future outbreaks. Given its properties, tea tree oil is also recommended for rashes, burns and wounds. Cucumber juice mixed with a few dashes of tea tree oil works as a great aftershave lotion for men.

Since tea tree oil wards off fungus, it is also used during pedicures, if the feet are cracked or riddled with ringworms.

Tea tree oil is good for the hair, and cures itching, persistent dandruff, and head lice. Simply massage a few dashes in, leave on for 5 minutes, then rinse the hair with a herbal shampoo and conditioner. Results will be evident with time.

Tomato

Tomatoes hold the goodness of vitamins A, B1, B2, B3, B5, B6, K, along with magnesium, iron and phosphorous.

Tomato juice is food for the skin. A natural astringent, it helps treat and prevent acne, shrinks open pores and regulates the secretion of sebum. Moreover, it fades tanning, and fights skin discolouration.

Tomato juice is full of antioxidants, so it helps combat free radicals in the body.

Turmeric

Turmeric is known for its anti-inflammatory, antibacterial and therapeutic properties. Hence, it helps treat acne, reduce inflammation and prevent breakouts. It also controls excessive secretion of oil by the skin's sebaceous glands. A face pack of turmeric powder, sandalwood powder and lemon juice is especially useful if addressing zits!

40

Turmeric fights pigmentation, lightens tans and fades scars. It is for this reason that it is often smeared across the body of a bride a day before her wedding, so she gets glowing, spotless skin! Interestingly, turmeric also inhibits hair growth, when applied regularly to the face and body.

Being an excellent exfoliating agent, turmeric can help eliminate signs of ageing.

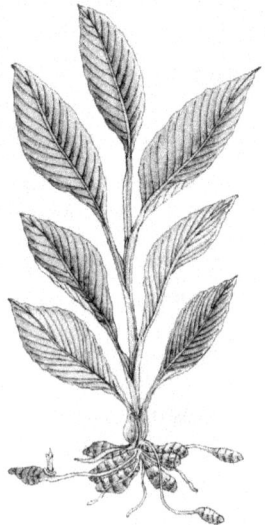

U

Urad Bean (Black Gram)

Urad beans are excellent for facial and hair care, since they are packed with vitamin B6, potassium and iron.

Urad beans have antimicrobial properties. They can therefore be used to combat acne. Simply mix a tablespoon of sandalwood paste and an equal amount of urad beans paste with rosewater. Dab this over acne spots, wash off after 10 minutes, and watch them heal! You'll be left with soft, flawless skin. If mixed with turmeric, urad beans not only fight acne but also stem facial hair growth.

Urad beans help address tans, and soothe sunburns. Ground urad beans mixed with curd lightens the complexion!

Finally, urad beans are good for the hair, and are often recommended to those suffering from alopecia.

W

Walnut

Walnuts are endowed with vitamin B6, magnesium, iron, copper and omega-3 fatty acids.

As a result, these dry fruits keep the skin youthful. The copper in them wipes off wrinkles and improves skin elasticity. The omega-3 fatty acids simultaneously lock in moisture and leave the skin hydrated. Moreover, since walnuts are packed with antioxidants, they combat free radicals and toxins and keep the skin youthful.

The nourishing fats in walnuts also fight skin inflammation. Walnut oil, for this reason, is also recommended for the scalp, if it is irritated. Further, walnut powder could be added to henna to add shine and nourish your hair with antioxidants.

Wheat Bran

Wheat bran is rich in vitamins B6 and E, besides minerals like iron.

Wheat bran is a natural exfoliant. When dead cells accumulate on the surface of the skin, it looks dull and lacklustre. At such points, a wheat gram scrub rids the body of old skin and makes it look youthful and fresh.

When mixed with other ingredients, wheat bran helps soften and nourish the skin.

42

Wheatgrass

Rich in vitamins A, B-complex, C, E and K, besides minerals like calcium, phosphorus and selenium, wheatgrass is excellent for the skin and hair.

Wheatgrass powder is an exceptional cleanser. It exfoliates, scrubs off dead cells, and revives tissue. Being a natural detoxifier, it rids the skin of external pollutants, and lends a glow to the body.

Consequently, wheatgrass powder also stems zits. Simply mixing wheatgrass powder and milk controls the spread of acne!

Wheatgrass combats the ageing process! It curbs the damage of free radicals. Further, it prevents the sagging of skin and promotes skin elasticity.

Wheatgrass is also known for its antiseptic properties. It treats rashes, burns and wounds, and soothes sunburnt skin.

Finally, wheatgrass powder is excellent for the hair. It addresses dandruff and scalp itchiness, and curbs premature greying.

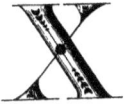

X

Xigua / Watermelon

Watermelons are rich in vitamins A and C, iron, magnesium, manganese and amino acids. They hold 6 per cent sugar and 92 per cent water.

Given the high water content in watermelons, they are natural moisturisers. Besides, their cooling properties make them an ideal cure for sunburn. Grandmothers often suggest mixing the juices of cucumber and watermelons, and dabbing the mixture over sun-damaged skin!

Watermelons are natural astringents and can be used as toners. Mix watermelon juice and honey if you have dry skin and need to tone. Both honey and watermelon will hydrate your face and leave it glowing!

Interestingly, watermelons also cure acne problems. Dab a cotton pod in watermelon juice and massage it across your cleansed face. Rinse off with cold water. With time, the size of your pores will diminish, your face will produce less oil, and the pimples will naturally heal.

Watermelons have antioxidants such as lycopene, which combat free radicals and fight the physical signs of ageing. Regular application of watermelon juice to the face irons out wrinkles and fine lines.

Ylang-Ylang

Ylang-ylang, or the flower of flowers, cultivated in Java, Sumatra and Madagascar, offers a sweet smelling essential oil. This oil holds linalool, caryophyllene and other aromatic components.

When applied topically, ylang-ylang oil suits both oily and dry skin types, for it balances sebum production. It also soothes, which is why it is often used in tropical islands to treat insect bites!

Ylang-ylang is known to benefit the hair by stimulating growth. Besides, it is believed to treat head lice.

However, this wonderful oil is best known for the effect it has on the nervous system. It eases stress, tension and fear, and bestows one with a sense of wellbeing and joy. Given its soothing effect, and the vital connection between happiness and health, ylang-ylang oil is often recommended for glowing skin and healthy hair.

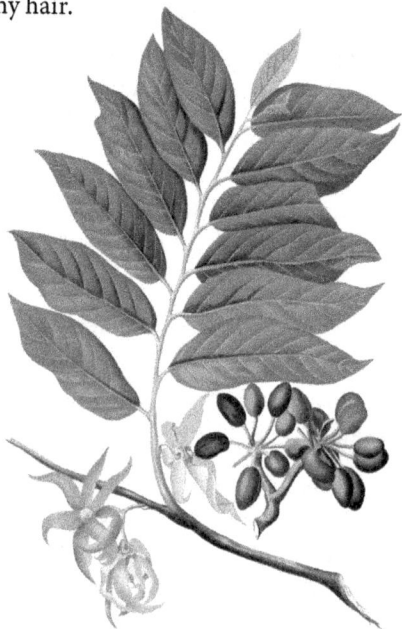

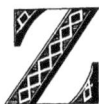

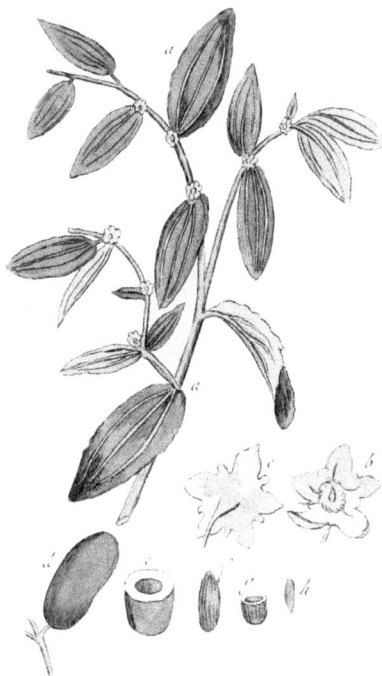

Z

Zizyphus (Ber)

The ber is filled with the goodness of vitamins B6 and C; it also has reserves of calcium and magnesium.

It is known to be antioxidant-rich. When applied to the skin therefore, it fights free radical damage, irons out fine lines, and keeps the face wrinkle-free. The ber is nature's anti-ageing solution!

The ber has anti-inflammatory properties too. Chinese medicine has long used ber extracts to treat redness, sunburns, and dryness. In India, the leaves are used to treat mouth disorders. Just boil the leaves with some salt, gargle well, and your gums will stop bleeding. Indians also use ber leaves to attend to stubborn boils. Merely grind ber leaves, and apply the paste to the boil-infested areas. The boils will vanish with time.

Finally, the ber leaf is food for the hair, and prevents greying.

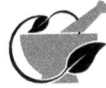

Skin Care
Introduction

The skin is the largest organ in the human body. It plays a vital role in protecting us against pathogens, and preventing excessive water loss. It also regulates our temperature and aids with the synthesis of vitamin D.

What is the Skin Made Of?

Every beauty book offers you skin facts, but often the approach is intimidating.

The fact is, the skin looks like a sandwich with 3 different layers – the epidermis, the dermis and the hyperdermis.

The epidermis is made of hardened cells which protect the inner layer; the hardened cells of the epidemis shed off when they die. These are replaced by new cells.

In the bed of the dermis are blood vessels, hair follicles, sweat glands. More importantly, the sebaceous glands are found here, and these govern facial skin.

The hyperdermis contains loose connective tissue, lobules of fat, and larger blood vessels than those found in the dermis.

Now, the lay person rarely concerns herself with the skin's composition. But knowing is important, so the right decisions can be taken. In my early years as a beautician concerned with the top layer of the skin, I tried applying a whole lot of packs on my face to observe the results. What intrigued me was this – the juices I applied often disappeared. The skin, I saw, had great receptive qualities and took in everything that was applied to it.

If this be the case, if the skin indeed eats, isn't it essential to feed it everything that's good? Isn't it imperative to offer it the best, like we would choose the healthiest of items to satiate our stomachs? To feed the skin the right meal, one must know it, understand its type and preferences.

What do we mean by skin type? We mean that your skin could be dry, or oily, or sensitive, or you could have combination skin. Or you could be blessed with normal skin.

Babies are generally born with normal skin. But today because expecting mothers opt for excessive medication, and have deficiencies, stress and improper eating habits, babies are born with dry, flaky or scaly skin. The truth is, the gift of good skin starts before your birth. It begins in your mother's womb.

What Does the Skin Want?

Our genes determine our physical attributes; we can't do very much to alter our genetic makeup. But what we can do is nurture and nourish ourselves, so we have better looking skin and hair.

Here are some prerequisites for healthy skin and hair.

Oxygen
We breathe without being aware of it; often, we breathe incorrectly. This damages the quality of our skin. We need

to be aware of our breathing practice; we also need to embrace the right techniques through breathing exercises like pranayama. This will ensure that fresh oxygen reaches the cells beneath the skin.

Though the skin receives most of the oxygen through the blood stream, it also takes some in through its pores. Constantly covering the skin with creams and lotions blocks oxygen intake.

Finally, we need to breathe in fresh air. We must avoid extremely polluted spaces, whenever possible, and use air conditioners and coolers minimally.

Sleep
Sound and peaceful sleep is a sure beautifying agent. Sleep for at least 8 hours at night, and follow a regular rhythm.

Equally, cleansing the face before sleeping is enormously important.

Water
The skin loves water. Water keeps the skin supple and hydrated. Along with adequate water intake – at least 8 glasses a day – one can also pamper the skin by drinking fresh vegetable and fruit juices and tender coconut water.

Food
Now that we know our skin laps up everything put on it, we ought to nourish it with all that is safe. Would you eat the ingredients listed in creams or lotions? Why would you feed the skin what the stomach would refuse?

Since time immemorial, women have used fruits, flowers, herbs and seeds to beautify themselves; this is a tradition we need to revive.

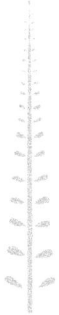

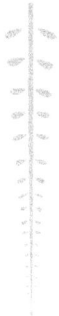

The skin also reflects what we eat. Therefore we need a rich and healthy diet, with fruits, leafy and green vegetables, whole grains, dry fruit seeds and nuts, and unrefined and cold pressed oils.

Peace

Our state of mind is conveyed through our skin. Being relaxed and peaceful will release hormones that keep the skin supple and young.

How Does One Care for the Skin?

Cleansing forms a crucial step in any beauty regime. For years, cleansing milk has been popular; it is believed that it clears the face of grime and dirt.

In the local pharmacy, one will find cleansing milk without an ounce of milk; the label is wholly misleading. We will find a range of face washes and soaps with umpteen promises, but with very little to offer in concrete terms. Soaps and face washes make the skin alkaline, rob it of whatever natural moisture it has. It is best to avoid them.

One needs to look towards nature. The best aspect of natural cleansers is that they offer multiple benefits.

You could cleanse your face with milk or curd. The milk not only cleans but also helps brighten the skin.

You could also cleanse with cucumber juice. It not only makes the skin dirt-free, but also brightens it and controls wrinkles.

I personally have never applied soap on my face, but simply use gram flour with turmeric. This not only keeps the skin fresh for hours but also grants it an undeniable glow.

Nature has blessed us with various cleansers in fruits and vegetables. Every fruit or vegetable has moisturising and toning effects when directly massaged onto the skin.

So going back to the age old rule of cleanse- tone-moisturise, a single fruit or vegetable could provide all these benefits. So easy, yet so very effective!

Coconut milk is an amazing example of a 3-in-1. Let's look at the recipe, shall we?

RECIPE TO CLEANSE-TONE-MOISTURISE

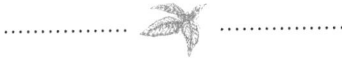

.... 🌿 ....

The Coconut Milk Mantra

Ingredient

20 dashes coconut milk

Method

Dip a cotton ball in coconut milk.

Use this as a cleanser to wipe off the dirt.

Massage a portion of it with gentle strokes, and rinse with water, which helps tone and moisturise.

This can be done twice daily.

....

How Does One Care for the Neck?

Allow your neck to contribute to the beauty to those necklaces!

Skin care is not restricted to the face alone. Most women miss out on pampering their neck while taking care of their face.

Remember: When you look after your neck, you tend to your face as well! A huge difference is seen in the texture of the neck and face, when the neck is tended to.

All the recipes in this book place an emphasis on applying packs not only to the face but also to the neck.

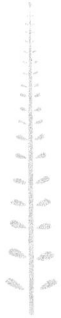

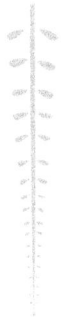

Common Skin Problems

ACNE

A single pimple or a boil can scare a 12-year-old or send a teenager scurrying for shelter in her room. It's not unusual for young boys and girls to lock themselves away from family and friends while battling acne, and try in vain to get the pimple off the face! The truth is, acne can impair social interaction, sometimes severely. Embarrassment can fast spiral into depression.

Acne afflicts both teenagers and those significantly older. It generally begins at puberty due to hormonal imbalances, and can continue to any age. Adult acne isn't at all uncommon.

Acne is an inflammatory condition. Overactive sebaceous glands, blocked hair follicles and clogged pores due to excess sebum production attract bacteria. This results in boils.

Why are some people more acne-prone than others? The most prominent reason could be genetic, and hormonal imbalances worsen the problem. Equally, improper eating habits, a diet rich in sugar or saturated fats, a deficiency in dietary fibre (which leads to irregular bowel movements), inadequate water intake, the absence of fruits and vegetables, a faulty cleansing of the face all contribute to acne. Finally, dandruff can trigger a spate of acne.

Treatment for Acne

There are some basic rules that can help you get rid of facial acne.

Do

❀ Cleanse the face with natural products.

❀ Keep the scalp free from dandruff.

❀ Drink plenty of water and consume fresh fruit juices.

❀ Eat plenty of fruits and fresh vegetables. Salads are strongly recommended.

❀ Practise breathing exercises and work out the body to improve blood circulation.

❀ Relax.

❀ Sleep for 7 to 8 hours daily.

Don't

❀ Consume sugar, white flour, and fried food items.

❀ Consume dairy products.

❀ Eat shell fish, prawns and seafood in general.

❀ Additionally, do apply the face packs that follow on a regular basis.

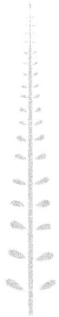

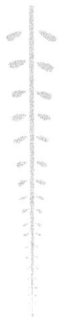

RECIESE TO COMBAT ACNE

....

Green Pack

Ingredients

4 margosa (neem) leaves

10 mint leaves

½ cucumber

Method

Wash the ingredients thoroughly in lukewarm water.

Grind the ingredients in a blender to form a smooth paste.

Apply the paste on acne.

Let it remain on the skin for about 5 minutes.

Wash off with cold water.

The pack can be applied twice daily.

....

All Spice Pack

Ingredients

2 tsp green gram lentil powder

¼ tsp turmeric powder

¼ tsp sandalwood powder

1 pinch clove powder

10 dashes cucumber juice or water

Method

Mix green gram lentil, turmeric, sandalwood and clove powder with water or cucumber juice.

Apply all over the face and neck. Avoid the eyes and the area directly around them.

Wash off pack after 5 minutes with cold water.

The pack can be applied twice daily.

....

Aromatic Pack

Ingredients

¼ cup apple cider vinegar

2 dashes tea tree oil

2 dashes lavender oil

2 dashes margosa (neem) oil

Note: This pack is suitable for those who are allergic to powders and pastes. Apple cider however needs to be tested on a patch of skin, before liberal application.

Method

Mix the ingredients and store the concoction in a glass bottle.

Shake the bottle well before using.

Apply with cotton-wool.

The concoction can be used 2 to 3 times daily

This blend can be stored for 2 to 3 days.

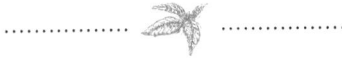

....

Marigold Spot Pack

Ingredients

15 marigold petals

4 margosa (neem) leaves

½ cucumber

½ cup coriander leaves

Method

Wash the ingredients thoroughly in lukewarm water.

Grind the marigold petals and coriander leaves in a blender to a smooth paste.

Apply the paste evenly over the troubled spots of acne.

Wash it off with water after 10 minutes.

Repeat the process twice daily.

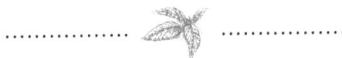

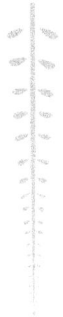

Holy Pack

Ingredients

15 holy basil (tulsi) leaves

1 tsp triphala powder

1 tsp red sandalwood powder

Method

Grind the holy basil leaves in a mortar with a pestle, till they become a thick paste.

Add the triphala powder and sandalwood powder.

Mix the ingredients.

Apply the pack on the face and neck. Avoid the eyes and the areas around them.

Wash off the pack with water after 5-10 minutes.

PIGMENTATION

Pigmentation is a fairly widespread skin problem. Although not as painful as acne, it does pose a more obstinate challenge.

How does one identify the problem? It is fairly obvious. If one's skin seems patchy – and especially if the patches are dark – it is a sign of pigmentation.

A harsh summer and exposure to heat is a common cause for pigmentation. But such discolouration of the skin can also occur due to a variety of other reasons, including hereditary factors, deficiencies, the use of spurious cosmetics, excessive bleaching and hormonal imbalances.

Pigmentation cannot be completely eradicated, but can be reduced considerably or controlled.

Treatment for Pigmentation

If treating pigmentation with natural products, you should be patient and consistent in adhering to the treatment. Simultaneously you must try taking the following measures.

- As far as possible, avoid the afternoon sun.

- Apply some protective cream even while cooking.

- Steer clear of poor quality beauty products.

- Stop bleaching completely.

- Avoid excessive use of chemicals on skin and hair. (Did you know that colouring your hair can contribute to pigmentation?)

RECIPES TO ADDRESS PIGMENTATION
AND DISCOLOURATION

Oatmeal Pack

Ingredients	Method
2 tsp almond powder	Mix the above ingredients, except the cucumber juice, to form a paste of applicable consistency.
2 tsp oatmeal powder	
½ tsp wild turmeric powder	
10 dashes milk or curd	Apply this on the pigmented areas.
½ cup cucumber juice	
	Wash off after 5 minutes with cucumber juice and then water.
	Ideally, apply the pack twice a day.

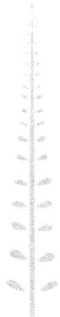

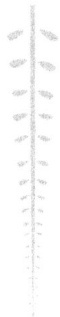

Coconut Magic

Ingredients

¼ cup grated coconut

¼ cup pistachios

Method

Grind the 2 ingredients into a smooth paste.

Massage this paste on the pigmented area for 5 minutes. Those with acne or boils need not massage, but simply dab the pack on.

Leave the pack on for 5-10 minutes, then wash it off with water.

Apply the pack twice daily.

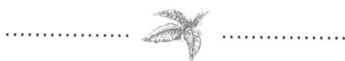

Scrub Pack

Ingredients

2 tsp green gram

2 tsp yellow gram

¼ tsp turmeric powder

10 dashes buttermilk

Method

Soak the above ingredients in buttermilk for 1 hour.

Next, grind them all into a paste.

Apply this paste across the face and neck in case of excessive pigmentation, or just over pigmented spots.

Wash the pack off with water after 10 minutes.

Apply twice daily for best results.

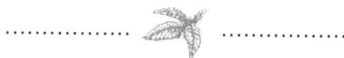

Vitamin A Pack

Ingredients

4 tsp carrot juice

4 tsp almond powder

4 tsp coconut milk

Method

Mix all the ingredients to form a paste.

Apply the paste on the pigmented parts.

Wash it off with water after 5-10 minutes.

Apply the pack twice daily till the pigmentation reduces.

....

Divine Juice

Ingredients

4 tsp coconut milk

4 tsp almond milk

2 tsp almond oil

2 dashes saffron oil

Method

Blend all the ingredients in a glass container.

Apply the mixture to the pigmented areas.

Wash it off with water after 10 minutes.

Use the mixture 2 to 3 times a day, and regularly.

This pack is extremely good for those with dry skin.

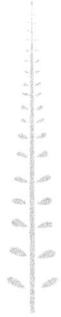

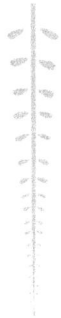

ROSACEA

Have you noticed your cheeks remaining red for extended periods of time?

No, you aren't blushing. And you aren't love-struck either.

If your cheeks and the areas surrounding them become red often or remain red, it is a call for attention. For you could be suffering from a chronic condition of the skin: rosacea.

This troubled state of skin normally affects those above the age of 30. It is primarily characterised by redness of the nose and the cheeks, with visible blood vessels, at times like bumps and small boils, and swelling. Often the skin feels very warm and tingles. The eyes could also turn red and watery or dry. If not attended to with the right products and at the right time, rosacea could become a semi-permanent or a permanent skin condition.

There aren't definite proven causes, but yes, there are some triggers with can aggravate the condition. Excessive intake of tea and coffee, extreme exercises, cosmetics are known to set off rosacea. Interestingly, while sunburn could spark off rosacea, cold winds or a cold and dry winter could also cause this skin condition.

One of the biggest culprits though is to be found beyond the ambit of diet and climatic conditions. During my early years of practice, I had a client. She was 36-years-old, and had rosacea: redness of cheeks with tiny bumps that had emerged over 6 months. The main triggers – sun, coffee, intense exercise routines, cosmetics – did not apply to her. She travelled only in enclosed cars, consumed minimal amounts of coffee, had a relaxed exercise regime, and used little or no makeup. I met her around August – in the middle of the grey Indian monsoons – so this could not be a case of accidental sunburn either. I was definitely concerned, since my packs, which normally bring stellar results, did not work to their maximum efficiency. It was then that I had a chat with her, to understand if there had been changes in her lifestyle. During the course of the conversation, she told me that she was going through various medical procedures to conceive, and that she was facing a lot of stress.

This then was the culprit! Emotional stress is one of the cruellest villains, and can aggravate rosacea. On my advice, my client started meditation, yoga and spa sessions that helped her relax. Once she began to de-stress, her rosacea automatically came under control.

Treatment for Rosacea

The following are recommended solutions for controlling rosacea.

- Treat the skin very gently. Do not rub or massage. After washing the face, wipe it with a soft cotton cloth. It is advisable to avoid Turkish towels, or rough material that could irritate the skin. No scrubs should be used.

- Cleanse with either an oatmeal soap or an aloe vera based soap.

- Drink plenty of water, tender coconut or fruit juices.

- Consume foods rich in beta carotene, vitamin B and C, zinc, and essential fatty acids.

- Flax seeds, rich in omega-3 and omega-6 fatty acids, should be made part of your diet. Foods and beverages that contain antioxidants – green tea, chamomile tea, and salads with apple cedar vinegar – can also help.

- Wear good sunglasses, and hats with broad brims, and apply a sandalwood based sunscreen, if you are required to travel in the sun.

- Stay relaxed and composed, so your skin breathes healthily.

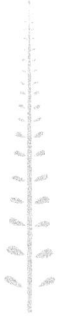

✿ Avoid dishes that are extremely pungent; use fewer spices in your meals.

Over the last 21 years, I have found that natural ingredients and fresh packs work wonders on rosacea. It is, of course, a very stubborn condition of the skin, yet with a little patience and a stringent regime, clients can get relief.

RECIPES TO ADDRESS ROSACEA

....

Zinc Pack

Ingredients

2 tsp oatmeal flour

2 tsp + ½ cup cucumber juice

1 crushed zinc tablet

Method

Mix the zinc tablet in 2 tablespoons of cucumber juice until it dissolves.

Add oatmeal flour to this solution and stir till it forms a paste.

Apply the paste on the affected areas.

Wash the pack off after 5 minutes with half a cup of cucumber juice and then water.

....

Fruit Cider Pack

Ingredients

4 tsp orange juice

1 tsp apple cider vinegar

2 tsp oatmeal powder

½ cup cucumber juice

Method

Mix all the ingredients except the cucumber juice, to form a paste.

Apply the paste on the affected areas.

Wash off after 5 minutes with cucumber juice and then water.

....

Aloe Pack

Ingredients

4 tsp aloe vera juice

4 tsp + ½ cup cucumber juice

2 tsp oatmeal powder

2 dashes lavender oil

Method

Mix all the ingredients, except the half-filled cup of cucumber juice.

Apply the paste on the affected parts.

Wash off with the half-filled cup of cucumber juice and then some water after 5-10 minutes.

Washing your face with buttermilk, tender coconut water or green tea water helps.

....

DARK CIRCLES

Dark circles are self-explanatory; they are shadowy patches around the eyes.

They are viewed as major eye disasters – unbecoming even on the prettiest of faces – since they tend to make one look old, akin to 'zombies'.

The truth is, dark circles are not merely aesthetically unappealing. They could also act as signals for a lurking health condition.

Under-eye dark circles could be caused by deficiencies, especially of vitamin B12 and iron. They could also get aggravated by poor sleep, nasal congestion, improper diet, excess salt intake and stress. Dark circles also have genetic links, and sometimes are directly linked to eye strain, due to excessive use of computers.

The condition spares nobody, and dark circles afflict both men and women, and sometimes – though not commonly – even children. The aged are also victims, because with age,

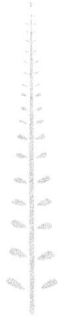

the skin loses its elasticity and collagen, becoming thinner and susceptible to dark circles.

Your eyes are amongst your most attractive features; with a little care, they can enhance your beauty considerably!

Treatment for Dark Circles

Those young, or those crossing 30, should take a few precautions to avoid dark circles.

- Take small breaks away the computer screen to help the eyes relax.

- Vegetable compresses, such as cucumber, can also be used at intervals to cool and relieve the area around the eyes. In fact, as you apply a cucumber cool compress, save some to eat!

- The best part of all natural treatments is that they work internally and externally. Consume diuretic foods like watermelons and celery that flush out excess water, reducing puffiness.

- Water is your elixir! Drink plenty of water to rebalance the fluids in your body, which in turn will help your dark circles fade.

- Irritants such as cigarette smoke or dust – which trigger the release of chemicals in the body to dilute the aggravating substance, and consequently enlarge blood vessels – also tend to cause dark circles. Try inhabiting non-smoking, pollution-free areas.

- Excessive use of eye makeup or poor makeup removal methods should be avoided.

Dark circles aren't easy to get rid of. But with constant care, you can definitely lighten them. And over a period of time, you can bid goodbye to them altogether.

RECIPES TO ADDRESS DARK CIRCLES

················ 🌿 ················

Oatmeal-Cucumber Eye Brightener

Ingredients

2 tsp grated potato juice

2 tsp grated cucumber juice

2 tsp oatmeal powder

1 tsp almond oil

Method

Mix all the ingredients together.

Dab 2 cotton pods in the solution.

Lie down and leave each cotton pod on your eyes for 5 minutes.

Remove the pods, and notice the difference!

················ 🌿 ················

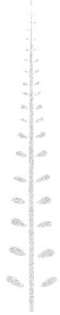

Cucumber Cool Compress

Ingredients

2 tsp grated cucumber

2 tsp grated potato

1 tsp vitamin E oil

Method

Mix all the ingredients.

Press the mixture over cotton pods.

Place these pods on the eyes for 5 to 10 minutes.

Once you remove the compress, eliminate all traces of oil with a cotton pod soaked in milk and cucumber juice.

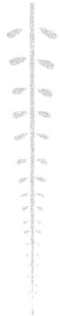

················ 🌿 ················

Simple Potato Magic

Ingredients

2 tsp grated potato

2 tbsp milk

2 tbsp cucumber juice

Method

Press grated potatoes on the cotton pods.

Place these pods on the eyes for 5 minutes.

Once you remove the pods, wash your eyes with a cotton pod soaked in milk and cucumber.

Alternatively

Raw potato juice can be applied over the eyes to reduce puffiness and dark circles.

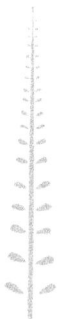

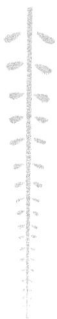

Lip Care

Our lips are often hidden under the cover of lipstick; indeed, most women feel half-dressed without gloss. Painted lips are a definite mood booster. As a result, a lot of time and money gets spent on the lips.

But what our lips demand is a simple, 5 minute, natural routine of care. They need softening and protecting just as regularly as the rest of the face.

Care for the Lips

There are some basic lifestyle decisions that ensure that your lips stay picture perfect.

- If your lips are chapping or peeling, or if they are excessively dry, make sure you increase your intake of vitamin B food items.

- Indulge in wheat germ, pearl millet (bajra), barley, lotus stems, raisins, almonds, papaya, jackfruits, pineapples, lettuce, cauliflowers, sprouted seeds, and oatmeal.

- Also, nothing is safer than applying edible natural products which help heal lips without side effects.

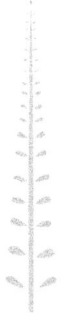

RECIPES TO NURTURE THE LIPS

Do you feel as though your lips are dry? Here is a recipe to make your lips soft and supple.

....

Vegetable Lip Softener

Ingredients	Method
2 tsp pumpkin paste	Mix all the ingredients together.
2 tsp coconut cream	
1 tsp honey	Chill the paste in a freezer for 10 minutes.
	Apply the paste 2 to 3 a day on the lips.

....

Do your lips look dull and tired? Here is a paste that will grant them brightness!

Fruit Lip Salve

Ingredients	Method
1 tsp dry almond powder	Mix all the ingredients together till they form a paste.
1 tsp papaya pulp	
1 tsp honey	Apply this paste on the lips using brush-like strokes. This acts as a gentle exfoliant, removing all peeled skin to give way to fresh skin on the lips.

....

Do you feel as though your lips are tanned and unflattering? Would you like to lighten them? Let almond and coconut come to the rescue.

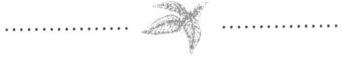

Coconut-Almond Touch

Ingredients	Method
2 tsp almond milk	Mix all the ingredients to collect the curdled milk.
2 tsp coconut milk	
1 tsp apricot oil	Chill the mixture.
1 dash lemon	Use the mixture twice daily.
	'Coconut-Almond Touch' will last for a period of 2 days if stored in the deep freezer.

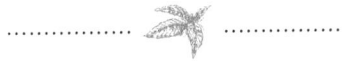

Finally, do your lips need pampering? Try this 100 per cent natural balm, which not only provides you with natural vitamins, but also grants you a lip smacking treat!

Pick-Me-Up Balm

Ingredients	Method
2 tsp strawberry pulp	Mix the ingredients till they form a paste.
2 tsp honey	
	Apply the paste on your lips.

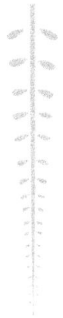

Back Care

There was a time when the back was one of the most neglected parts of the body. This could be because we assumed that nobody could see its flaws. It could also be because we did not get to observe it closely, like we could the face.

However, today's fashion trends – with low cut blouses and halter-necks – encourage us to flaunt our backs. A clean back then becomes mandatory. Where earlier we had to focus on those aspects that were visible – the face or the lips – the times we live in demand meticulous and careful attention to the body as a whole.

In this regard, we often come across statements like: 'It's difficult to maintain a beautiful back, especially with the hectic routines we have!' But the truth is: All it takes is a few simple natural procedures... and we are certain to find ourselves with the backs we desire!

Common Dermatological Problems Associated with the Back

What makes us feel self-conscious about our backs? The answer is simple – pimples, boils, rashes, blemishes and pigmentation.

The causes for these could be hereditary or hormonal factors. But there are other causes too such as dandruff, constipation and improper diet, and often, improper cleansing or neglect, poor use of cosmetic products, and/or allergies to certain synthetic products.

Here are some natural remedies for your back.

Treatment for Dermatological Problems Associated with the Back

There are a few simple routines that will ensure that our backs are clean and smooth.

- Clean the back effectively on a daily basis.

- Try using a loofah for the back while having a bath, since it helps with exfoliation.

- While out in the sun, protect your back with an umbrella or cover it well with a cotton scarf or dupatta.

- Change your shirt regularly, especially if it gets sweaty.

- Eat food items that are high in antioxidants, like fruits, vegetables and whole grains.

- Reduce stress levels, for when you worry, your adrenal glands produce excessive cortisol, and this makes your sebaceous glands produce extra oil.

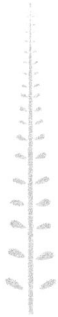

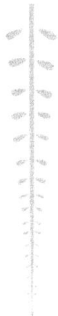

RECIPES TO ADDRESS DERMATOLOGICAL PROBLEMS ASSOCIATED WITH THE BACK

ACNE AND BLEMISHES

To get rid of your 'bacne' – spots and blemishes on the back – a paste made of green gram needs to be applied regularly.

....

Green Gram Back Mixture

Ingredients	Method
1 cup green gram	Grind the green gram well.
2 tsp sandalwood paste	To this, add the sandalwood, holy basil and marigold paste.
2 tsp holy basil (tulsi) paste	
2 tsp marigold paste	
1 tsp wild turmeric powder	Now add the wild tumeric powder.
	Mix all the ingredients well till they form a paste.
	Apply the paste on your back like a mask.
	Wait till it dries and then rinse it off with water.

PIGMENTATION

Pigmentation of the back is often caused by hormonal changes, hereditary factory, health issues (like liver disorders), and extensive bleaching. If a parent has pigmented skin, then there is a possibility of the child inheriting the same problem.

A natural mixture that helps battle back pigmentation uses the strengths of almond and oatmeal. It should be used regularly.

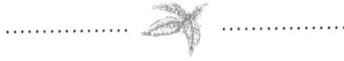

....

Almond-Oatmeal Back Mixture

Ingredients	Method
½ cup almond powder	Mix all the ingredients together till they form a paste.
¼ cup oatmeal powder	
1 tsp turmeric paste	Apply the paste on your back like a mask.
1 tsp khus khus paste	
1 tsp papaya paste	Wait till it dries and then rinse it off with water.
1 tsp cucumber juice	

This mixture keeps the back smooth and shiny back by creating an acidic layer on the skin and warding off bacterial attacks.

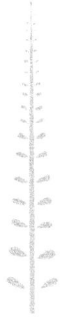

EXFOLIATION

The back needs regular exfoliation so it remains spotless. The 'gentle fruit exfoliator' and the 'lentil scrub' are perfect in this regard.

....

Gentle Fruit Exfoliator

Ingredients

1 cup raw papaya paste

½ cup apple paste

¼ cup honey

½ cup milk

Method

Mix the ingredients, except the milk, till they form a paste.

Rub this gentle pack on the back with massaging strokes for 5 to 10 minutes.

Wash the pack off with milk and then lukewarm water.

....

Lentil Back Scrub

Ingredients

¼ cup red lentils (masoor dal)

¼ cup almond

¼ cup green gram

½ cup milk or papaya paste

Method

Grind the red lentils, almonds and green gram, so they attain a coarse consistency.

Mix this with papaya paste or just milk to scrub the back for 10 minutes.

Wash it off with water after 5 minutes.

....

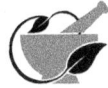

Hair Care

Introduction

There isn't a poem describing a woman's beauty that doesn't mention her long, lustrous hair. Hair and attractiveness have been synonymous from time immemorial.

Indeed, hair is a marker of good looks not just for women but also for men. As our understanding of fashion and style evolves, men have started placing an emphasis on the quality of their hair, not least because hair – its presence or absence – acts as a sign of age. A bald, grey-haired man can appear far older than he is, and can seem as though he is 40 even if he is in his mid-20s.

The beauty market is crowded with umpteen ads for a variety of hair products. Beauty clinics too promise hair replacement and hair growth at exorbitant rates.

But the fact is that a little care from the very beginning, and with the right natural products, will ensure that your hair is healthy. While your genes play a huge role in deciding your hair volume, growth, and extent of greying, the general health of your hair is in your hands.

What is the Hair Made Of?

Hair is made up of the same protein found in human skin, teeth and nails. This protein is called keratin and is composed of amino acids and cysteine disulphides. Their levels and structure determine how your hair looks.

The hair grows from follicles within the skin. The part of the hair inside the follicle is known as the hair root and the part outside is known as the shaft. At the base of the hair root is a bulb which uses the nutrients it receives to form cells. It is vital that you feed the bulb with natural ingredients like herbs, fruits and vegetables, as this will help it prepare healthy new cells.

You may well ask: Why feed the bulb natural ingredients? Well, it's quite simple. Your body ingests natural ingredients in the form of food, and distributes the nutrients across your body. If these very natural ingredients are applied externally, our body soaks them in too! It is easy for the body to accept familiar ingredients. Hence the motto: Go natural!

What Does the Hair Want?

As with the skin, the quality of your hair mirrors your inner health. If you go on a vigorous diet, or neglect your diet, the consequences are borne by your skin and hair, and they reflect your lifestyle switch.

Here are some prerequisites for healthy hair.

A Balanced Diet
To have healthy hair, a balanced diet comprising vitamins A and B, calcium, silica, iron and zinc, proteins and essential fatty acids is vital.

No Smoking
Normal blood circulation keeps your follicles alive.

Smoking leads to a drop in blood circulation, which leads to an increase in hair fall.

Relaxation

Stress is not good for your health in general, and your hair often gets directly affected by nervous tension. A strand of healthy hair typically goes through 3 phases: the active phase, when it grows; a transitional phase, when it stops growing; and the final phase, when it is wholly at rest, following which it sheds in the course of a normal day. A traumatic life situation can push much of your hair directly into the third phase – the rest phase – causing it to shed prematurely. This is the body's way of coping, of taking a breather, while coming to terms with an anxiety-ridden life change. For the general health of your hair, therefore, it is important to practise yoga or mediate, or keep time aside to simply relax, so no matter the challenges you confront, you remain calm.

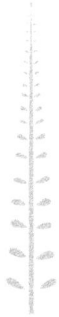

Sleep

Adequate sleep, for at least 8 hours every night, is imperative. When you're asleep, your hair goes through a period of repair and regeneration. Without sufficient sleep, your hair loses its lustre and bounce.

Regular Hair Care

The hair asks for nurturing, and a regular hair-care regime is essential for healthy locks.

How Does One Care for the Hair?

Oiling

Hair requires food internally and externally. Oiling is a vital external hair care measure, since it improves circulation through massage. The choice of oil is entirely personal – the oil could be made of olive, coconut, sesame, castor, mustard or almond.

My choice of oil would be a combination of pure virgin coconut oil, castor oil with a small amount of sesame oil. Mixing this with herbs, plants and flowers like Indian pennywort (Brahmi), fenugreek (methi), curry leaves, margosa (neem) and hibiscus helps strengthen the hair and nourish the scalp.

Washing and Shampooing
Chemical shampoos strip the oil from your hair, thus making it dry and unmanageable. They are also alkaline in nature.

When washing, always wet your hair thoroughly before applying shampoo. You must take care to rinse out every bit of the shampoo before drying out your hair.

To restore the natural pH balance of your hair, add 2 teaspoons of apple cider vinegar to a mug of water, and rinse your hair with this.

Conditioning
For those with dry and brittle hair, pre-conditioning before shampooing is recommended. Those with normal hair can condition after shampooing.

To condition the hair, rub a dash of either rosemary oil, or lavender, or ylang ylang on your palms and apply this on wet hair.

Drying with Care
Taking care of your hair when wet is essential. Never brush hair when it is damp. Once dry, try combing the hair layer by layer from its ends, moving upwards. This ensures that the tangles are removed easily without damaging the hair.

Common Hair Problems

PREMATURE GREYING

People colour their hair for a variety of reasons – because they are bored with the present condition of their hair, for novelty, or because they wish to experiment. But the most common reason is this: to conceal premature greys.

What leads to premature greying? Well, a combination of various internal and external factors. Genetics, lack of melanin, vitamin B deficiency, extensive use of chemicals, hair styling treatments, strong shampoos, internal and external heat, stress all contribute to premature greying.

Age too is a determinant. Once you hit your 30s, your hair follicles slow down the process of producing melanin, which is the pigment that determines the colour of your hair.

Treatment for Premature Greying
There are some basic rules that can help delay the appearance of greys.

❀ Avoid using chemical colours and harsh synthetic products on your hair.

❀ If you must camouflage grey hair, make use of nature's own treasures – for instance, henna – instead of opting for chemical colours.

❀ Protect your hair during summer while walking outdoors, by either wearing a wide hat or by wrapping a scarf around your hair.

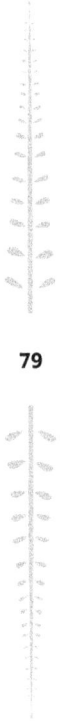

✿ Constantly keep your hair nourished by applying the juices of vegetables, herbs and dry fruits.

✿ Eat food rich in vitamins B and C, copper, iodine and iron.

✿ Adopt relaxation techniques.

A consistent effort in doing this will help control greying to a great extent.

RECIPES TO ADDRESS PREMATURE GREYING

There are a few excellent receipts that address problems like premature greying. In all cases, washing your hair with cold water helps prevent greying.

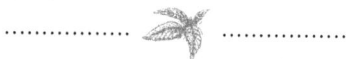

....

Indian Gooseberry Pack

To prevent premature greying, massage the scalp for 5 to 10 minutes with extra virgin coconut oil and castor oil, mixed with a dash of fresh amla juice.

Following this, an Indian gooseberry pack from the following ingredients needs to be applied.

Ingredients	Method
4 tbsp Indian gooseberry (amla) powder	Mix the ingredients together till they form a paste.
2 tsp Indian pennywort (Brahmi) powder	
4 tbsp fenugreek (methi) powder	Apply the pack on the scalp and hair.
½ cup coconut milk, freshly extracted and thick	Leave this on for 20 minutes.
	Wash with a mild herbal shampoo.

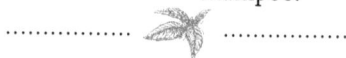

....

Herb Juice

Ingredients

¼ cup margosa (neem) juice

¼ cup fresh Indian gooseberry (amla) juice

¼ cup fresh coconut milk

¼ cup wheatgrass juice

Method

Mix all the 4 juices together.

Massage this mixture onto the scalp for about 5 minutes.

Tie up the hair and put on a shower cap.

Wash off the juice with a mild herbal shampoo after about 20-25 minutes. Use a conditioner too.

Apply this 4 times a week.

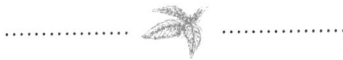

Indian Gooseberry Magic

Ingredients

½ cup dry grated coconut

½ cup fresh grated coconut

1 cup fresh curry leaves

6-7 Indian gooseberries (amla) cut into small pieces

½ cup water

Method

Soak the Indian gooseberries in water overnight.

The next day, mix all the ingredients.

Grind into a coarse rough paste and then extract the juice, which should be greasy in texture.

Massage this into the scalp and hair.

Wash off with a herbal shampoo after 20-25 minutes.

Apply twice a week for best results.

Prepare a fresh potion every week.

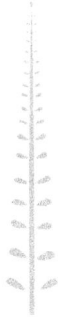

Colouring Hair

Greying is a huge source of anxiety for both men and women.

Since time immemorial, henna has been used to dye the greys. It not only colours, but also helps with hair cell growth, and protects. Indeed, henna is a safer choice than chemical dyes. It also fades less swiftly.

However, it is important to remember that henna leaves, when powdered and used, dry the hair. This is doubly so when herbs are used. Equally, henna addresses uneven greys, but it does not suit those who have entirely grey hair. This is because, while the red tinge of henna isn't obvious when uneven white strands get coloured, it becomes glaringly apparent when a white mop of hair becomes a blazing orange.

Since henna dries the hair, it should be mixed with fruits and dry fruits, so it conditions the hair and does not make it brittle.

Let me share with you my secret henna recipe.

RECIPE FOR COLOURING HAIR NATURALLY

....

Henna and Hair

Ingredients

2 cups henna leaves

6 Indian gooseberries (amla), cut into small pieces

¼ cup fresh coconut

¼ cup beet slices

2 tsp coffee

Method

Wash the henna leaves and semi-dry them.

Now grind the rest of the ingredients together and extract a juice. Add the juice to the ground henna leaves for a smooth henna paste.

Application

Partition the hair into several segments, and apply the henna paste to each segment.

Start with the roots, and apply to the remaining length of hair.

Wind each segment, and twist it, as the paste is applied.

Ensure that each partition attended to is closest to the segment just completed.

Continue this process, till all your hair has a layer of henna paste, and is piled up.

Cover your head with a shower cap.

Leave the henna paste on for about 2 hours, or longer if you'd like a deeper tint.

Wash off with cold water.

Henna paste can be stored for a maximum of 2 days.

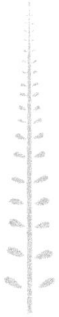

....

Dealing with Chemical Dyes

83

I must admit that hair looks gorgeous with colouring and other styling techniques. But do we know the price that we are paying by opting for chemical dyes?

The truth is, chemically dyeing the hair is always a bad idea. Not only do chemical dyes make the hair dry and frizzy, but they also set a precedent for more greying. As a result, once you start chemically dyeing your hair, there is no end in sight!

If used continuously, chemical colours can bring out the worst in your hair, and can make strands brittle, weak and unattractive. While those blessed by their genes can survive harsh chemical colours, the rest end up with damaged tresses, or worse thinning hair.

I understand the pressures that people face daily to look youthful and attractive. For many, henna is not an option, and for still others, flawlessly coloured hair is vital for professional and personal reasons.

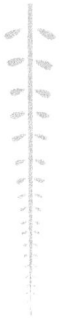

What we need to aim for in such cases is a middle path, a balance. We need to take care of hair the natural way. It is a matter of simple logistics. Colour is one chemical, mass produced shampoos are another, and chemical conditioners are a third. Opt for one chemical, at the very most, at any given time. Therefore if you choose to chemically colour your hair, use only natural shampoos and conditioners. This will restrict the damage to your scalp.

I would recommend using the bounties of nature, to gift your hair with the goodness it has been denied after a chemical procedure.

RECIPE TO BALANCE AND TREAT COLOURED HAIR

Fruit and Egg Hair Food

Ingredients

1 banana, cut into slices

1 slice ripe papaya, cut

¼ cup oil (olive or sesame or almond)

¼ cup thick coconut milk

2 egg yolks

2 dashes lavender oil

Method

Grind all the ingredients in a mixer into a smooth paste.

As in the case of henna, partition the hair, apply the paste to the length of each segment, and twist each section.

Tie the hair into a neat bun and cover it with a shower cap.

Wash the hair after 20 minutes with an aloe vera based shampoo and conditioner.

Apply this hair food twice a week for nourished locks.

HAIR FALL

It is altogether distressing when we find several broken strands of hair on our comb.

Hair fall is a common enough problem, and the reasons for it could be vary. Improper diet, stress, nervous tension, lack of sleep, deficiencies, thyroid and hormonal imbalances, and the excessive use of chemical products could all contribute to the loss of hair.

Treatment for Hair Fall

Here are some precautions you can take to combat hair fall.

- Improve your diet. Make sure you include proteins, iron and vitamin B rich food items.
- Resort to yoga and meditation to relieve yourself of stress.
- Sleep for at least 7 to 8 hours.
- Avoid exposing your hair to chemical treatment. This includes styling, blow drying and ironing.
- The regular application of herbs, fruits and vegetable juices on your scalp and hair nourishes and strengthens the roots from within.
- Wash your hair with cold water.
- While drying your locks, avoid rubbing, as rubbing can weaken hair follicles.
- Comb your hair gently and patiently.

If you are losing hair, massage your scalp each morning. This will stimulate your blood vessels. If your hair is dry, opt for almond or olive oil. However, if you have oily hair, avoid oil altogether as the condition could get far worse.

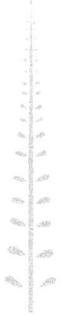

Apart from this, here are a couple of recipes that will do wonders for your hair problem! Always remember to massage your hair with oil (if you have dry hair) before applying these homemade potions.

RECIPES TO ADDRESS HAIR FALL

....

Fantastic Fenugreek

Ingredients

2 tablets brewer's yeast, crushed into a fine powder

15 fenugreek (methi) leaves

10 curry leaves

2 tbsp sesame seeds, soaked overnight

4 tsp fenugreek (methi) seeds, soaked overnight

Method

Grind all the ingredients together, and extract a thick lotion.

Now massage the extracted lotion into your scalp and hair.

Wash this after 30 minutes with cold water.

Use a mild herbal shampoo and conditioner.

Follow this ritual thrice a week for best results.

Flower Power

Ingredients	Method
5 red hibiscus flowers	Grind the petals of the hibiscus flowers with the other ingredients.
¼ cup fenugreek (methi) seeds, soaked overnight	
¼ cup curry leaves	Extract the lotion with a sieve.
¼ cup fresh coconut	Massage this into the scalp.
	After 10 minutes, wash it off with cold water.
	Use a mild herbal shampoo and conditioner.

....

DANDRUFF

Dandruff is an infection of the sebaceous glands and results in the scaling and itching of the scalp.

What causes dandruff? There are several triggers – stress, excessive use of chemical shampoos which strip the scalp of natural oils, and contact with someone suffering from the condition. Additionally, climatic conditions too are known to affect the scalp.

Excessive scratching of the scalp can result in secondary hair disorders, which is just one of the reasons why dandruff must be controlled as soon as possible.

Treatment for Dandruff

Here are some precautions you can take to battle dandruff.

❀ Make sure your scalp and hair are always clean by washing your hair 3 times a week with a mild herbal shampoo and conditioner.

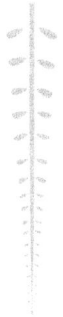

🌿 Keep your hair tied to avoid secondary skin disorders like acne on the face and back.

🌿 Use your own combs and hair accessories, and keep them clean.

🌿 Follow a healthy diet, and indulge in vitamin B enriched food items. Avoid oily, fried food.

🌿 Drink at least 8 glasses of water a day.

🌿 Relax. Stress is known to cause dandruff.

🌿 Massage your hair regularly with some coconut milk and neem juice. Apart from this, here are some kitchen recipes to treat the hair problem.

RECIPES TO ADDRESS DANDRUFF

Beet Blend

Ingredients

¼ cup beet juice

¼ cup coconut milk

¼ cup curd

3 tsp olive oil

Method

Blend all the ingredients, including the beet juice (which reduces stickiness and dandruff).

Massage the juice into the scalp.

After 15 minutes, wash off with cold water, a mild herbal shampoo and conditioner.

In case of stubborn dandruff, repeat twice a week.

Beet-n-Neem Juice

Ingredients

1 tsp margosa (neem) juice

¼ cup coconut or olive oil

¼ cup beetroot juice

Method

Mix the margosa juice (which takes away dandruff's itchiness) and the oil.

Massage the combination into your scalp for 10 minutes.

Next apply and massage beetroot juice to the scalp and rest of your hair.

After 20 minutes, shampoo and condition with a mild herbal product.

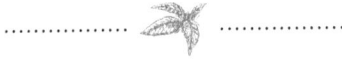

....

Apple Cider Last Rinse

It is important to follow this recipe for a last rinse.

Ingredients

4 tbsp apple cider vinegar

2 dashes tea tree oil

1 cup water

Method

Mix all the ingredients together.

Rinse your hair with the solution twice a week.

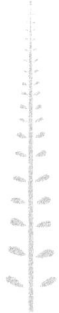

....

ALOPECIA

Hair loss in patches is known as alopecia.

Alopecia Areata is generally an auto immune disorder in which the hair follicles are attacked by the immune system, thereby causing hair loss in patches. The causes for alopecia could also be hyper- and hypo-thyroidism, or other hormonal imbalances. Alopecia could also be caused by the use of steroids, low iron and vitamin levels, and sudden stress or depression. Further, the excessive use of chemical colours or heat induced styling procedures can lead to hair loss in patches.

There are different kinds of alopecia, and these are differentiated based on the pattern of balding.

Treatment for Alopecia

Here are some precautions you can take every day to control alopecia.

- A good nutritious diet is essential to control alopecia internally. Adding kelp, the outer skin of potatoes, peppers, cucumbers (rich in silica) to your diet could boost your immune system, thereby controlling alopecia. Other food items that improve your immunity are berries, kale, pomegranate, coconuts, mushrooms, green tea, garlic and spices like turmeric and cinnamon. Traditionally fermented fare, vitamin C rich food items, and a zinc rich diet with oysters and beans can help one fight alopecia. Omega-3 fatty acids are also recommended.

- Relax. Stress can strain your immune system and cause alopecia.

- Go natural. Use only herbal products that are free of toxins.

Apart from this, there are some quick and easy recipes that can help with alopecia.

RECIPES TO ADDRESS ALOPECIA

Castor Care

Ingredients

3 tbsp castor oil

3 tbsp mustard seed oil

5 tbsp coconut milk

Method

Mix all the ingredients together.

Massage this into your scalp and across the length of your hair.

Leave overnight and wash it off the next day with a mild herbal shampoo and conditioner.

Apply twice a week at least to restart hair growth.

Onion Wash

Ingredients

½ onion

5 fresh aloe vera leaves

10 tbsp mustard seed oil

Method

Grind the onion till you get a pulp.

Grind the pulp of the aloe vera leaves to get a cup of fresh juice.

Mix both the pulp and the juice with the mustard oil.

Apply the solution to the bald patches.

Wash off with cold water, and with a herbal shampoo and conditioner, after 20 minutes.

Apply twice a week to stimulate hair growth.

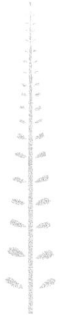

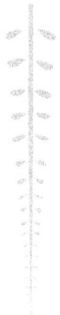

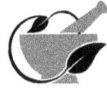

Beauty & Seasons
Introduction

As the seasons drift and change, your skin, hair and body care regime also must. In a country like India especially, where topographies vary, where climatic conditions shift month after month, the health of your skin and hair is linked to the vagaries of sun, wind, rain and snow.

Although your genes define your skin and hair type, the seasons influence their texture. While every skin and hair type is unique, and each person reacts to passing seasons differently, there are certain precautions everyone can take to keep his or her body healthy.

Over the last 21 years of analysing skin and hair, I have come to see that skin and hair problems often correspond to the drift of seasons: spring, summer, monsoons and winter. Summers and winters, with their extreme climatic conditions, take a toll on the skin and hair. Monsoons act as a welcome relief for the face, but are a definite no-no for the hair, hands and feet. Spring is the happiest season for many reasons, but also because your skin and hair see rejuvenation and regrowth. Spring therefore is when you can really revive yourself after the harsh dryness of the winter and before the cruel heat of summers.

Here's to getting your skin and hair ready for all seasons!

Spring

Spring in India starts in March, after a dry, cold winter. Spring marks the start of festivals from Sankranthi to Holi and Easter, before summer takes over.

Spring gives the body time to recuperative after the assault of winter. It is also when the body learns to prepare itself for an unforgiving summer. In spring therefore, one must take especial effort to ensure that the skin and hair are healthy, well maintained, glowing with health and joy.

94

SKIN CARE

There are some easy, undemanding rituals that grant perfect skin. Here is a list of recommendations, all natural and toxin-free, so you have a spring in your step!

Drinking Liquids
Drink plenty of water or consume fresh fruit juices. A prerequisite for good skin, these hydrate the body, reduce fluid retention and lessen puffiness.

A Healthy Diet
The skin acts as a barometer of internal health. It is important to follow a diet of whole grain food items, fresh vegetables and fruits. Try brown bread, oats, brown rice, pearl millet (bajra), sorghum (jowar), wheatgerm, barley, carrot, beetroot, red and yellow pepper, parsley, tomato, lotus stems, spinach, pumpkin, cucumber and soya bean. Also include fruits like avocado, orange, apple, banana, cherry, and grapes.

Natural Care
Feed your face. 60 per cent of everything applied on the skin enters your body, so why not apply something edible? Look through your kitchen shelves to find a whole range of beauty products like lentils which act as cleansers, dry fruits like almonds which brighten and nourish the skin, herbs like holy basil and sandalwood which cool the body, fruits like papaya and banana which act as softeners, or honey which moisturises.

Gentle Nurturing
Be gentle while washing, massaging or scrubbing the face. Avoid extremes of very cold or very hot water.

Makeup-Free Sleep
Remove all traces of makeup before retiring to bed. Let your skin breathe.

Rest
Sleep well. Sleep helps the skin rejuvenate. Cut down on your sleep and you'll find your skin looking dull.

Pursuing Happiness
Finally, stay happy. A good mood brings a glow to the skin. Happiness is best makeup artist and a joyful smile on the face goes a long way towards making one attractive. Negative thoughts like jealousy, sadness, anger create unhealthy enzymes in the body, and mar inner radiance.

Spring Cleansers

Dry Skin
Almond milk, coconut milk and apricot oil can be individually used as natural cleansers.

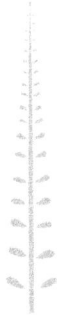

RECIPE TO CLEANSE DRY SKIN

················ ················

Wheat Bran Cleanser

Ingredients

3 tsp olive oil

3 tsp wheat bran

Method

Mix the 2 ingredients together to form a paste.

Apply the paste across the face and neck, with gentle massaging strokes.

After 5-10 minutes, wash this with cold water.

Apply daily for best results.

················

96

Oily Skin

Buttermilk and honey act as excellent cleansers for those with oily skin.

RECIPE TO CLEANSE OILY SKIN

················ ················

Lime-n-Milk Cleanser

Ingredients

3 dashes lime

3 tbsp milk

Method

Mix the 2 ingredients together to form a solution.

Apply the solution across the face and neck, with gentle massaging strokes.

After 5-10 minutes, wash this with cold water.

Apply daily for best results.

················

Spring Moisturisers

No matter your skin type, it is important to moisturise the skin regularly. A homemade moisturiser can be whipped up with some fairly basic ingredients.

RECIPE TO MOISTURISE ALL SKIN TYPES

.... *️ ....

Lettuce Moisturiser

Ingredients	Method
2 tsp lettuce juice	Mix all the ingredients together to form a paste.
½ tsp almond oil	
½ tsp oatmeal powder	Apply the paste across the face and neck, with gentle massaging strokes.
½ tsp honey	
	After 5-10 minutes, wash this with cold water.
	Apply daily for best results.

....

Spring Facial Masks

You may have cleansed and moisturised your face, but there is a final beauty ritual that is recommended: the use of facial masks. Facial masks provide deep nourishment to the skin, by detoxifying it and increasing blood circulation.

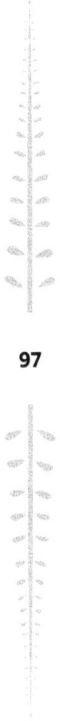

RECIPE FOR A SPRING FACIAL MASK

....

Spring Fruit Mask

Ingredients	Method
2 tsp orange juice	Mix all the ingredients together to form a paste.
2 tsp watermelon juice	
2 tsp bran	Apply the paste across the face and neck, with gentle massaging strokes.
	After 5-10 minutes, wash this with cold water.
	Apply daily for best results.

....

SPRING CARE FOR HANDS AND FEET

Your hands and feet disclose your age when your face doesn't. One therefore cannot afford to ignore them.

The simplest trick to get great hands and feet is this: using what remains of a face pack you have just made, or a cream, on a regular basis. However there are other recipes that address issues specific to either the hands or the feet.

Tanned Hands and Feet

Do your hands and feet appear unevenly suntanned? It must be sunshine, and it must be spring. Here are a few quick-fix solutions.

RECIPE TO ADDRESS TANNED HANDS AND FEET

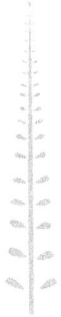

Lime-n-Orange Hand-n-Foot Pack

Ingredients	Method
1 bowl green gram flour	Mix all the ingredients, till you get a paste.
½ cup oats	Apply the paste on the hands and feet.
½ cup lime juice	Wash off with cold water after 10-15 minutes.
½ cup orange juice	Apply daily for best results.

Tired, Cracked Feet

Spring makes the world look beautiful. Spring is also when we wander, to explore countries and continents. However, the end result is that we have tired and cracked feet.

RECIPE TO ADDRESS TIRED, CRACKED FEET

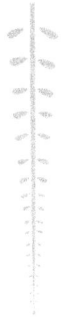

Herbal Foot Spa

Ingredients

2 lime slices

5-6 margosa (neem) leaves

5-6 mint leaves

5-6 rose petals

2 tbsp rock salt

2 dashes pine oil

2 dashes lavender oil

Method

Fill a pedicure tub with warm water.

Boil the margosa and mint leaves, and lime slices, and filter the solution.

Add this solution to the water in the tub.

Crush the rose petals and add them in.

Add the rock salt, pine and lavender oil.

Soak your feet in this mixture for at least 20 minutes, while seated in a relaxing chair.

Follow this daily for excellent results.

....

HAIR CARE

There are some easy steps that grant one perfect hair. Here is a list of suggestions, natural and toxin-free, so you have lustrous locks in spring!

- Avoid exposure to the sun, even if it is only spring, chlorinated water, areas with high levels of pollution, and rooms with air conditioning.

- Avoid yo-yo diets and other improper forms of weight control. Eat healthy. Gorge on those spring fruits.

- Sleep, and relax.

- Check for thyroid problems if confronted with excessive hair loss.

- If you have oily hair, opt for a good, dry scalp massage for about 4 minutes, without the use of oil. If you have dry hair, opt for a massage with almond or olive oil. If you are losing hair, make sure that you massage your scalp each morning before your hair wash, to stimulate the blood vessels.

- Select your shampoo and conditioner according to your hair type. Go for a moisturising shampoo and conditioner if your hair and scalp are dry. If they are oily, opt for cleansing ones. Don't undermine the use of conditioner. While shampoos are for the scalp, conditioners are for your hair.

❀ In spring, shampoo your hair on alternate days, and condition it after every wash.

❀ Use either cold or lukewarm water to wash and rinse your hair, as hot water tends to weaken the roots.

❀ For dry, chemically-treated or damaged hair, towel dry and apply 2 to 3 drops of serum (available at salons) and leave on. This provides extra nourishment, shine and gloss to the hair, prevents breakage, tackles frizz and creates tangle-free tresses.

❀ While brushing or combing your hair, remain gentle and patient. If you comb your hair very roughly, you might lose those precious strands of hair.

❀ While drying, do not rub the hair. This will weaken the follicle and make the hair brittle and dull.

❀ Get a regular trim to avoid split ends.

❀ Yes, we know spring is the time to experiment, but avoid changing your hairstyle drastically on a regular basis.

Spring Hair Food

Once spring announces its arrival, it's time to begin feeding your scalp with natural ingredients. This guarantees excellent results.

Dry Hair
If your hair is excessively dry, here's an excellent natural recipe.

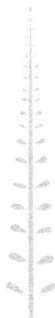

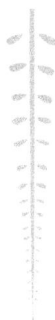

RECITE TO ADDRESS DRY HAIR IN SPRING

....

Papaya Hair Food

Ingredients

½ cup papaya paste

1 egg

½ cup thick, fresh coconut milk

4 tsp coconut oil

2 dashes lavender, rosemary or ylang ylang essential oil

Method

Beat the egg into the papaya paste.

Now add the coconut milk, and mix.

Place the contents in a glass bowl and add one of the essential oils. You now have a ready-to-use paste.

Massage warm coconut oil into the scalp for 5 minutes.

Next, apply the paste on scalp.

Tie your hair up in a bun. Cover it with a shower cap.

After an hour, wash with cold water. Use a mild herbal shampoo and herbal conditioner.

Use this hair food at least once a week.

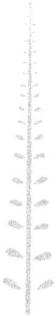

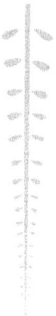

....

Oily Hair

If your hair is very oily, here's an excellent natural recipe.

RECIPE TO ADDRESS OILY HAIR IN SPRING

Fenugreek Hair Food

Ingredients

½ cup coconut water

15 fenugreek (methi) leaves

4-5 margosa (neem) leaves

2 egg whites

4 Indian gooseberries (amla)

15 curry leaves

Method

Wash the fenugreek, margosa and curry leaves thoroughly and cut them fine.

Cut the Indian gooseberries into small pieces.

Grind the fenugreek, margosa and curry leaves and the Indian gooseberries in a mixer with some coconut water, till you get a juice.

Beat the egg whites and add to the juice.

Massage the juice into scalp and hair for about 5 minutes.

Wash off with lukewarm water, and then with cool water.

Use at least once a week.

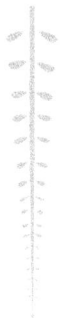

Summer

It's April. Summer's in, and so are the rising temperatures and sweaty days. The skin is instantly affected, as is the hair. Overexposure to the sun can lead to premature ageing of the skin, wrinkles, and dryness; it can also lead to bleached and damaged hair.

It therefore becomes especially important to follow a definite and regular regimen to ensure that your body remains healthy.

SUMMER SKIN CARE

There are some basic rituals that grant perfect summer skin. Here is a list of recommendations, to avoid summer skin woes!

- Increase your water intake substantially.

- Add fresh fruits and vegetables to your diet. These help with the process of natural exfoliation. They also ensure that the skin remains cool and less susceptible to ailments.

- Avoid the sun.

- If you must step out, apply a natural sunscreen.

- Over-exposure to the sun accelerates the ageing process. Try using moisturising creams and which have red sandalwood as their main ingredient, for this acts as sun protection.

❀ Ensure that you wear a hat, carry an umbrella or cover your head with a scarf, if outdoors.

❀ Apart from this, it is important to pamper the skin on your face, torso and feet.

SUMMER FACIAL CARE

Summer beings with it a number of conditions like acne, pimples, boils, heat boils, rosacea, excessive oiliness and hypersensitivity.

But perhaps the most common summer malady is tanning. This is the body's defence mechanism against the threat posed by the sun. Sunlight encourages the skin to step up the production of melanin, to prevent skin burns and the penetration of damaging rays. A lot of people get especially self-conscious when their face tans unevenly.

There are some natural kitchen recipes however that can come to the rescue, and help with tans, sun-dulled skin, sun burns, over-heated skin, heat boils, prickly heat boils and hypersensitivity.

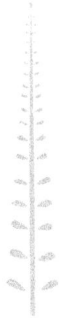

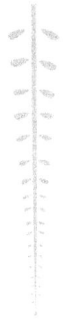

RECIPES TO ADDRESS FACIAL TANNING

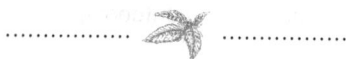

Summer Facial Tan Fighter

Ingredients

2 tsp curd

2 tsp almond powder

2 tsp green gram

1 tsp turmeric powder

Method

Mix all the ingredients to form a paste.

Apply across the face and neck twice daily.

Leave on till semi-dry, then rinse with water.

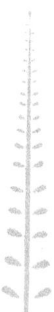

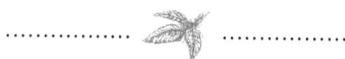

Buttermilk-n-Almond Facial Tan Fighter

Ingredients

4 almonds

3 tsp red lentils (masoor dal)

¼ cup buttermilk

Method

Soak the almonds and red lentils in buttermilk for 2 hours.

Next, grind these into a fine paste.

Apply evenly across the face and neck.

Wash off with some more buttermilk.

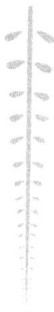

RECIPE TO ADDRESS SUN-DULLED FACIAL SKIN

....

Skin Glow Tonic

Ingredients

¼ cup watermelon juice

¼ cup orange juice

¼ cup carrot juice

1 tsp honey

1 dash lime

Method

Mix all the ingredients in a glass bottle.

Refrigerate for 5 minutes.

Apply this tonic all over face and neck.

Let it dry for 10 minutes.

Apply the second coat.

Let it also get absorbed by the skin for 10 minutes.

Now wash the face with lukewarm water, followed by cold water splashes.

Repeated application will supply the skin with vitamins, and the honey will help moisturise.

107

....

RECIPE TO ADDRESS FACIAL SUNBURN

....

Sunburn Face Pack

Ingredients

2 tsp hung curd

4 tsp watermelon juice

6 tsp soaked almond paste

Method

Mix all the ingredients to form a paste.

Apply this on the face and neck on returning home after a day out.

After 5-10 minutes, wash off with water. Your skin will be considerably brighter, cooler, less sore, and your tan will reduce.

....

RECIPES TO ADDRESS OVER-HEATED FACIAL SKIN

....

Summer Facial Coolant

Ingredients

½ cup oatmeal

¼ cup watermelon, grated

¼ cup cucumber, grated

Method

Mix all the ingredients to form a paste.

Apply a thick layer across your face and neck.

Wait for 5-10 minutes, before washing this pack off with water.

Apply twice daily.

Since this is an excellent refresher and coolant, those with heat boils and rashes will also benefit from this pack.

....

Summer Fruit Coolant

Ingredients

½ oranges, peeled

½ lemon

3 slices apples

4-5 grapes

1 slice watermelon

¼ cup oatmeal or chickpea flour.

Method

Grind all the ingredients together to form a paste.

Apply across the face and neck.

After 5-10 minutes, wash off with cool water.

Follow this ritual once daily.

This pack, apart from cooling and freshening the skin instantly, supplies it with natural vitamins.

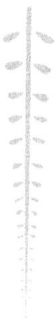

RECIPE TO ADDRESS FACIAL HEAT BOILS

················ ················

Summer Heat Boil Fighter

Ingredients	Method
10 holy basil (tulsi) leaves	Grind the ingredients to form a smooth paste.
10 mint leaves	
4 margosa (neem) leaves	Apply this paste on the heat boils twice or thrice a day.
	Wash off with water each time around after 5-10 minutes.
	Follow this ritual till the boils disappear.

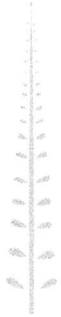

··

RECIPE TO ADDRESS FACIAL PRICKLY HEAT BOILS

················ ················

Prickly Heat Boil Fighter

Ingredient	Method
¼ cup buttermilk	Dab buttermilk on the boils twice or thrice a day.
	Wash off with water each time around after 5-10 minutes.
	Follow this ritual till the boils disappear.

··

RECIPES OF QUICK-N-EASY FACE MASKS, MASSAGES AND COOLANTS

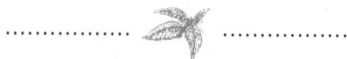

················ ················

Yoghurt Mask

Apply fresh curd (or buttermilk). It helps remove a tan and prevent sunburn.

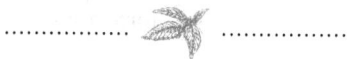

················ ················

Cucumber Mask

Just applying grated cucumber on the face and neck help cool the skin, besides acting as a natural astringent.

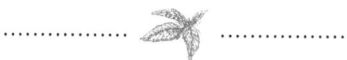

················ ················

Jojoba Massage

For face massages, use jojoba or plain coconut oil which is light and penetrating.

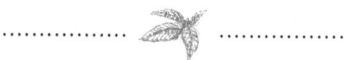

················ ················

Cool Waters

Spraying cold water (rosewater could be added) makes skin dewy fresh on a hot day.

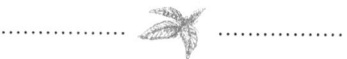

················ ················

Ice Magic

Ice cubes wrapped in a cling bag or a napkin make a wonderful de-bagger for puffy eyes and for a face puffed with water retention. This could also help circulation. (Please note: Those with very sensitive skin and/or with broken veins on the cheeks should not try this.)

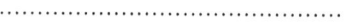

················

SUMMER EYE CARE

The windows of your soul and body need constant care in summer. It is important to wear glares when outdoors. On returning home, water rinses are also very useful. Simply try splashing some water to which fruit juice or rosewater is added. This will cool the eyes.

Apart from this, there are some easy recipes that can work wonders on summer-weary eyes.

RECIPE TO REDUCE EYE PUFFINESS

Summer Eye Mask

Ingredient

¼ cup grated cucumber (or wheatgrass paste)

Method

Close your eyes and place grated cucumber on them.

Sit back, and leave this on for 10 minutes.

Wipe off the shredded cucumber.

Apply twice daily to reduce puffiness and water retention.

111

RECIPE TO COOL THE EYES

Fruity Eye Mask

Ingredient

1 slice watermelon

Method

Extract the pulp of the watermelon.

Place this on a cotton pod.

Close your eyes, and cover them with the pod for 10 minutes.

Wash off with cool water.

The peels of bananas can also be placed on the eyes to cool them.

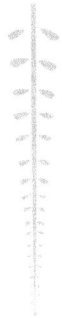

SUMMER BODY CARE

During summer, body massages help relax tired muscles. Herbs like Indian pennywort (brahmi) or essential oils like sandalwood help cool the entire body.

A small cup of apple cider vinegar added to a bucket of water can sooth itchy, flaky skin, and calm sunburn.

A bath is equally refreshing, especially if you dip into natural packs made of green gram paste mixed with mint and lemon, or sandalwood with buttermilk. These help cool the body, and also reduce some discolouration or uneven tans.

RECIPE TO COOL THE BODY

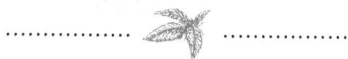

112

Cooling Summer Uptan

Ingredients

¼ cup sandalwood powder or paste

1 cup green gram powder

½ cup oatmeal powder

¼ cup margosa (neem) paste

¼ cup coriander leaves

1 cucumber, grated

¼ cup buttermilk

½ cup rosewater

Method

Mix the ingredients, except the rosewater, to form a paste.

Apply this paste all over the body.

Leave this on for 10 minutes.

Wash off with cool or lukewarm water.

Spray some rosewater all over the body.

Follow this daily for excellent results.

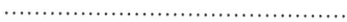

SUMMER FOOT CARE

The old technique of soaking the feet for 10 minutes is an effective way of relaxing and reviving them during summer. How exotic you want to make this ritual is left to you!

However, if you have no time for a foot bath, rub rosemary oil or diluted apple cider vinegar across your feet, massaging them for about 5 minutes before your bath.

If you suffer from foot odour, wear socks made of natural fibres so your feet can breathe. Avoid tight shoes. If you must wear tight shoes though, try sprinkling some sandalwood or chamomile powder into them. Once indoors, try to air your feet as frequently as possible.

In the meantime, here are some quick foot soaks for summer.

RECIPES TO ADDRESS SORE FEET

Herbal Foot Soak

Ingredients

5-6 margosa (neem) leaves

5-6 mint leaves

5-6 shredded marigold flowers

6 tbsp rosewater

2 dashes pine oil (optional)

Method

Take a vessel of hot water.

Add the margosa and mint leaves, shredded marigold flowers, and rosewater.

Keep stirring till you notice a little colour in the mixture.

Now fill a pedicure tub with lukewarm water.

Pour the entire mixture into the tub.

Add pine oil in case your feet ache.

Soak your feet in this for about 10 minutes.

Follow this twice a week for excellent results.

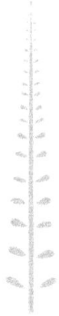

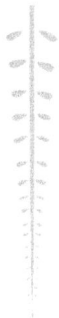

Sandalwood Foot Soak

Ingredients

3 dashes sandalwood oil

¼ cup sandalwood paste

2 cucumber slices

Method

Add the sandalwood oil to a bucket of water, full three-fourths of the way.

Soak your feet in this.

Relax by closing your eyes and placing cucumber slices on them.

After 5 minutes, extract your feet from the bucket.

Apply sandalwood paste on your feet.

After 15 minutes, when dry, place your feet back in bucket of water and wash off the paste.

Follow this every day for outstanding results.

....

SUMMER HAIR CARE

Any form of heat, be it internal or external, can destroy perfectly good hair. Hence, keeping the scalp cool during hot raging summers is a must.

There are some basic practices that grant perfect summer tresses. Here is a list of recommendations.

- Avoid blow drying your hair, or taking hot water hair baths.

- Carry an umbrella and a scarf to cover the head while outdoors.

- Hair really does grow faster in the summer, when a lot of it is in the growth stage. As a result, it is important to get regular trims to avoid split ends.

Applying an extract of herbs (like henna, Indian pennywort or brahmi, mint and aloe vera) and fruits helps cool the scalp and provides essential vitamins and minerals to the hair. While herbs may be a little drying for the scalp, mixing them with fruits balances their impact and helps soften the hair. Care however has to be taken while cleaning and grinding the herbs.

Apart from this, you can pamper your hair with some easy kitchen recipes!

RECIPE TO COOL THE SCALP

....

Herbal Hair Coolant

Ingredients

¼ cup Indian pennywort (brahmi) leaves

¼ cup margosa (neem) leaves

¼ cup mint leaves

4-5 hibiscus leaves

4 tbsp coconut water

Method

Grind all the leaves with coconut water, and extract a juice. (Plain water could be added but coconut water is more cooling.)

Massage this juice across the scalp and hair.

Rinse well after 10 minutes with a mild herbal shampoo and conditioner.

Apply thrice a week for excellent results.

Note: Those with coloured hair should not try this.

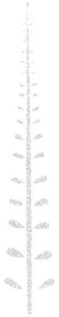

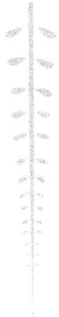

SUMMER RECIPES FOR COLOURED, CHEMICALLY TREATED HAIR

Those who have no option but to chemically colour or treat their hair should try using natural ingredients prior to and during shampooing and conditioning, at least once a week. This keeps your hair nourished and protected during harsh summers.

....

Coconut Hair Food

Ingredients

¼ cup fresh coconut milk

¼ cup aloe vera juice

1 slice papaya

1 banana

¼ cup milk

¼ cup castor oil

¼ cup coconut oil

Method

Mix the coconut and castor oil, and add a few dashes of coconut milk.

Massage your hair with this for 10 minutes, taking especial care to be gentle with coloured, chemically (and consequently dry) hair.

Mix the milk, aloe vera juice and a dash of coconut milk to form a tonic.

Massage this all across the hair and scalp and leave on for 20 minutes.

Now grind the papaya and banana to form a fruit pulp. Apply the fruit pack all over hair, especially the roots and the ends.

Wash off after 20 minutes using a mild herbal shampoo.

Condition the hair with some aloe vera gel.

Rinse with cool water.

Follow this ritual at least once a week.

....

Almond Hair Care

Ingredients

½ cup almond oil

½ cup papaya paste

½ cup milk

2 eggs

2 dashes ylang ylang essential oil

Method

Mix all the ingredients to form a mayonnaise like concoction.

Massage this into the scalp and hair.

After 10 to 15 minutes, wash off with a mild herbal shampoo and aloe vera conditioner.

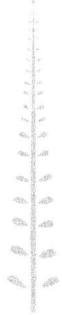

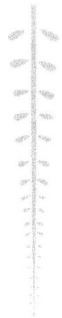

....

Monsoon

It's June, and the monsoons are close. It's when we choose to stay indoors, drink a hot cup of tea, and eat steaming bhajjias. However, this year, resolve to change old habits. Make this monsoon a season to pamper your hair and body.

Brew some soups that nourish the skin and tresses. Prepare freshly ground pastes for your face. And pamper your feet, so they remain healthy even after navigating mucky roads.

SKIN CARE

There are some basic rules to follow, so your skin glows during the monsoons!

- No matter how tempting, avoid deep-fried food items. Have a diet rich in raw vegetables and fruits, with vitamin C. Consume plenty of water.

- If you suffer from foot odour or excessively sweaty feet, include barley, parsley, lettuce, celery, cucumbers and sunflower seeds in your diet regime.

- Bathe in cool or lukewarm water.

- Wax the arms, underarms and legs to prevent infection.

- Many assume that sunscreens can be skipped during the monsoons. However, the sun's UV rays can penetrate through dense cloud cover, and cause skin damage. Always use sunscreen protection while outdoors during the monsoon.

❀ Avoid heavy makeup.

❀ Avoid high heels, which not only make you lose balance on slippery roads, but also cause back trouble.

❀ Fungal and bacterial infections are common during the rainy season, largely on account of damp skin. Keep the body dry at all times.

❀ Switch to cotton clothes as they allow the skin to breathe.

❀ Wear socks made from natural fibres, because they help the feet breathe and reduce perspiration. Peel off wet socks immediately.

❀ Dry your shoes daily even if they are waterproof.

❀ When working at a desk, remove all footwear to air the feet as frequently as possible.

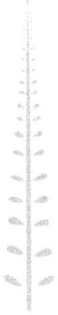

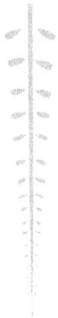

119

MONSOON FACIAL CARE

The humidity in the air during the monsoons can disturb the skin. There are some easy recipes that can help restore the balance.

RECIPE FOR A MONSOON FACE PACK

....

All-Skin-Types Monsoon Pack

Ingredients

¼ apple

¼ bananas

¼ cup oatmeal powder

¼ cup dry almond powder

1 tsp honey

¼ cup milk

¼ cup rosewater

Method

Blend the apple, bananas, oatmeal and almond powders, honey, and 3 teaspoons milk in a mixer to form a paste.

Apply this paste across the face and neck in massaging strokes.

After 5-10 minutes, wash off with the remaining milk.

Generously splash some chilled rosewater.

....

MONSOON FOOT CARE

The feet need especial care during the monsoons.

Nothing can be more embarrassing than dirty, cracked soles, after wading through muddied puddles of water. Worse, if we choose to wear closed shoes or gumboots, we are left with smelly feet!

Once the rains announce their arrival therefore, here are some rituals worth following.

- Scrub your feet daily using a pumice stone. Gently exfoliate, in small, circular motions, to remove stubborn patches of dry skin. Try rubbing husk and papaya paste to naturally exfoliate.

- Get a good foot massage weekly to help relax and aid circulation.

- Give yourself a regular pedicure, either at a reputed and clean salon or at home.

- Take a relaxing foot bath by adding essential oils like lavender, rosemary or sage. When you add essential oils to a foot soak, not only do your feet relax but your mind also calms down. After all, when the oils are mixed in warm water, they release aroma molecules which relax the mind and body. Note: If you suffer from asthma or have a history of respiratory problems, do not use essential oils unless you consult a doctor.

- Nurture your feet with foot masks made of almond powder, orange peels, milk, oats and lime.

RECIPE FOR A HOME PEDICURE

121

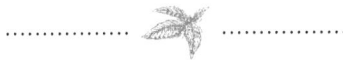

Marigold Pedicure

Ingredients

15-16 marigold petals

2 lime slices

2 tsp margosa (neem) juice

Herbal cream with cocoa butter

Equipment

A foot tub

Vegetable loofah

Foot scraper

Nail cutter

Nail filer

Buffer

Method

Fill the tub with warm water.

Add marigold petals, the slices of lime and the margosa juice.

Now soak your feet in the solution.

Rub the lemon slices in the tub across the length of your feet, and especially on cuts and cracks.

Use a food scraper to gently cleanse the soles and the heels.

Use the vegetable loofah to scrub and remove dead cells.

Remove your feet from the tub and wipe them clean and dry.

Cut or file the nails with the cutter and filer.

Use the buffer to add shine to your nails.

Take a generous helping of the herbal cream, mix it with a dash of water, and massage it across the soles and heels. Also massage it across your legs, right up to your knees.

If you have help, ask someone to take over the massage, so you can relax.

....

RECIPE TO ADDRESS RAIN-TIRED FEET

....

Aromatic Bath Soak

Ingredients

2 dashes lavender oil

2 dashes pine oil

2 dashes sandalwood oil

6-8 rose petals

Method

Fill a foot tub with warm water.

Mix all the ingredients in this.

Soak your feet in this blend for 10-15 minutes and relax.

Follow this ritual twice a week.

....

RECIPE TO ADDRESS FUNGAL INFECTIONS AND SWEATY FEET

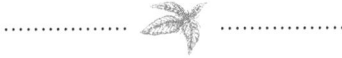

Tea Tree Oil Foot Cure

Ingredients

2 dashes tea tree oil

2 dashes geranium oil

2 dashes lemon grass oil

10 margosa (neem) leaves

Method

Heat the margosa leaves in water.

Pour this water into a tub.

Add the remaining ingredients.

Soak your feet in this mixture for 10-15 minutes and relax.

Follow this ritual twice a week for excellent results.

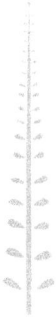

RECIPE TO ADDRESS DARKENED, DULLED FEET

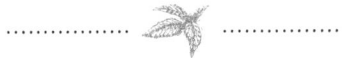

Almond Foot Care

Ingredients

½ cup red lentils (masoor dal) powder

½ cup almond powder

1 cup milk

2 tsp glycerine

Method

Mix the red lentils powder, almond powder, glycerine and the half cup of milk to form a paste.

Apply this paste across the feet and legs

After 10-15 minutes, when dry, rub the remaining half cup of milk all over.

Wash with lukewarm water.

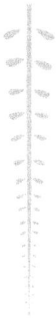

RECIPE TO ADDRESS CRACKED, HARDENED HEELS

....

Castor Oil Monsoon Foot Care

Ingredients

3 dashes castor oil

3 dashes olive oil

3 dashes coconut oil

2 tsp sugar

2 tsp lime

Method

Mix all the ingredients.

Massage the mixture into the skin of your feet, till the oils are completely absorbed.

Repeat twice a week.

....

MONSOON HAIR CARE

There are some basic rules to follow, so your hair remains healthy during the monsoons!

- Don't let your hair stay wet for a long time, or you could get a hair disorder.

- If outdoors, carry a small Turkish towel, so you can rub the dampness off the scalp and hair if caught in a downpour.

- Do not tie wet hair. Leave it untied till it dries.

- When at home, wash the hair with beetroot and neem juice.

- A common myth is that hair baths lead to a cold during the monsoons. This is far from true. Hair washing should continue as always to avoid hair loss. In fact, an unexpected holiday due to heavy showers gives you ample time to pamper your hair!

RECIPE FOR MONSOON HAIR CARE

There is one excellent recipe to solve multiple hair problems including limp hair, odour due to damp and wet hair, hair fall, loss of volume, and dandruff.

.... ~ ....

All-Purpose Monsoon Hair Pack

Ingredients

¼ cup almond oil (or any other oil of your choice)

½ cup thick coconut milk

¼ cup fenugreek (methi) seed extract

¼ cup milk

¼ cup aloe gel

2 egg yolks

2 egg whites

2 dashes rosemary oil

4 dashes lavender oil

4 tsp henna leaf powder (optional)

Method

Grind the milk, egg yolks, castor oil, fenugreek seed extract and coconut milk together.

Pour this ground mixture into a glass bowl.

Add 2 dashes of rosemary and lavender oil. As mentioned earlier, those with breathing difficulties or asthmatic conditions should avoid aromatic oils like lavender or rosemary.

Those with thin or limp hair could add henna leaf powder too. You now have a thick mixture.

For those who catch a cold easily, place the ground mixture in a bowl of warm water for some time.

Massage the scalp with the almond oil (or the oil of your choice), with gentle but firm strokes, for 5 to 7 minutes.

Now apply the thick, ground mixture into the scalp and hair.

Tie the hair in a knot or a bun with hair clips.

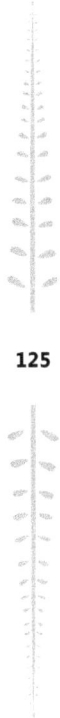

Put on a shower cap, to avoid stains down the nape.

After 10 minutes, wash the hair with lukewarm water.

Use a mild herbal shampoo.

Beat the egg whites into natural aloe gel, to get a foam-filled mixture.

Add the remaining 2 dashes of lavender oil to water.

Now wash the hair with the 2 solutions.

Follow this ritual once a week for healthy hair during the rainy season.

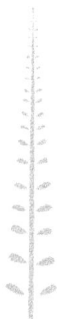

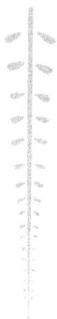

....

Winter

Come October and the temperature starts dropping in India. Winter is close. While it brings welcome relief from the singeing heat of summer, and the mugginess of the monsoons, it also wreaks havoc on the skin and hair.

To continue with your normal routine when the mercury drops simply means looking and feeling chapped. The lips, elbows, cheeks, feet protest! During the last months of the year, all our bodies need winter-proofing.

127

SKIN CARE

There are some basic rules to follow, so your skin survives the assault of winter.

❀ Moisturise! This cannot be stated often enough.

❀ While it is enticing jump into a hot shower, it is important to avoid the temptation. Use cool or lukewarm water.

❀ Pamper yourself with an oil bath.

❀ Pat your skin dry with a soft towel. Do not rub the skin.

❀ Ensure that all your skin products are alcohol-free. Alcohol strips away moisture.

❀ Flaxseed oil can moisturise your body from the inside, since it have reserves of vital fatty acids. Do include it in your diet.

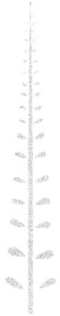

❀ Drink plenty of water, so your skin remains hydrated.

❀ Finally, do not lick your lips! This will only make them chap.

While moisturising, here are some points to bear in mind.

❀ Make sure you moisturise when skin is damp.

❀ Use a vitamin E moisturiser.

❀ Avoid applying soap before moisturising.

❀ Do not excessively wash the skin or hair.

❀ Should one moisturise before going to bed? Contrary to popular belief, the skin needs to breathe and repair itself at night, and moisturisers impair this process. All the skin needs at night is a very light lotion to prevent dehydration. If your skin feels dry, you could opt for extra moisturising during the day.

Winter Moisturisers

There are some natural moisturises that keep the skin youthful. Here are some quick, kitchen recipes for them:

RECIPE TO MOISTURISE DRY WINTER SKIN

....

Papaya Dry Skin Pack

Ingredients

2 tsp papaya paste

2 tsp almond paste

1 tsp vitamin E oil

2 tsp orange pulp

¼ cup milk

Method

Mix all the ingredients, except the milk, to form a paste.

Apply this across the face and neck.

After 10 minutes, wash off with milk.

Apply this daily for excellent results.

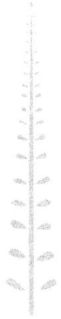

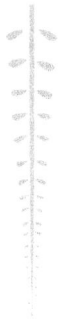

RECIPE TO MOISTURISE OILY WINTER SKIN

....

Jojoba Oily Skin Pack

Ingredients

2 tsp buttermilk

2 tsp jojoba oil

2 tsp water

Method

Mix all the ingredients together to form a paste.

Apply this across the face and neck.

After 10 minutes, wash off with lukewarm water.

Apply daily for excellent results.

Winter Cleansers

I would recommend avoiding soap. Soap robs whatever little natural moisture the skin holds. Instead try these recipes.

RECIPE TO CLEANSE DRY WINTER SKIN

.... 🌿 ....

Oatmeal Dry Skin Pack

Ingredients

¼ cup oatmeal flour

1 tsp vitamin E oil

1 tsp milk

Method

Mix all the ingredients together, to form a paste.

Apply this across the face and neck.

After 5-10 minutes, wash off the pack with lukewarm water.

If 2 tablespoons of milk and 2 dashes of vitamin E oil are added to the lukewarm water, the skin feels even suppler.

Apply daily for excellent results.

....

RECIPE TO CLEANSE OILY WINTER SKIN

.... 🌿 ....

Wheatgrass Oily Skin Pack

Ingredients

2 tsp green gram flour

2 tsp wheatgrass paste

1 tsp honey

1 tsp water

Method

Mix all the ingredients together to form a paste.

Apply this across the face and neck.

After 5-10 minutes, wash off with lukewarm water.

Apply daily for excellent results.

....

WINTER BODY CARE

When you wake up on winter mornings, the skin on your body is likely to feel tight and dry. It is asking to be fed with moisturising natural products!

RECIPE FOR A WINTER WASH

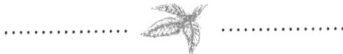

Lavender Oil Body Wash

Ingredient

2 dashes lavender oil

Method

Add the lavender oil to your bathing water, and have a bath.

Pat the skin dry very gently.

When the skin is still damp apply a natural moisturiser. You body will feel rejuvenated.

Follow this ritual daily for excellent results.

131

WINTER LIP CARE

Chapped lips are generally the first sign that winter is approaching. If your lips are excessively chapped or dry, check your intake of vitamin B food items. Feast on sprouts, vegetables, oats, wheat germ flour and yoghurt.

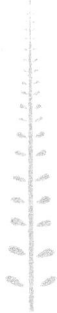

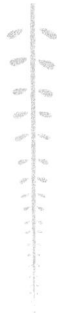

RECIPES FOR HEALTHY WINTER LIPS

....

Pumpkin Lip Balm

Ingredients

2 tsp pumpkin paste

2 tsp almond oil, naturally extracted, not perfumed

2 tsp milk

Method

Put all the ingredients in a blender and grind them.

Store the resultant pulp in a small bottle with a large mouth in the refrigerator, for up to a week.

Apply this pulp to the lips 2 to 3 times daily.

....

Orange Lip Moisturiser

Ingredients

8 sections orange

3 tbsp honey

4 apricots, soaked overnight and ground into a paste.

Method

Blend the ingredients well, to form a paste.

Store this in a glass bottle, in a refrigerator, for up to week.

Apply this paste on your lips 2 to 3 times daily.

RECIPES FOR WINTER LIP GLOSSES

Remember to avoid harsh lipsticks during winter. All the lipsticks you apply get consumed. It's time you swallowed something edible!

....

Natural Lip Gloss

Ingredients

2 tsp honey

2 tsp almond oil

2 tsp vitamin E oil

3 tsp strawberry pulp, sieved

Method

Blend the ingredients.

Store the resultant paste in a glass bottle, in a refrigerator or preferably the freezer, for up to a week.

Apply this paste to your lips 2 to 3 times daily.

....

Orange Lip Brightener

Ingredients

¼ cup orange pulp

¼ cup honey

Method

Blend in equal proportions.

Apply 2 to 3 times.

....

WINTER HANDS AND FEET CARE

Your hands and feet face the onslaught of winter. Feet are known to get cracked, while the hands get chapped and torn. There are some natural recipes that can come to the rescue.

RECIPES TO ADDRESS DRY, CRACKED FEET

. . . .

Honey Foot Spa

Ingredients

½ cup honey

¼ cup olive oil

1 tsp melted cocoa butter

Method

Take a tub or a bucket of warm water.

Mix all the ingredients in it with a large wooden spatula.

After washing your feet, soak them in the solution.

Keep rubbing your feet in the solution.

After 5 minutes, pat your feet dry.

. . . .

Honey Foot Cream

Ingredients

¼ cup olive or almond oil

1 tsp cocoa butter

1 tsp honey

2 tsp rosewater

Method

Collect all the ingredients, except the rosewater, in a container.

Place this container in an even larger vessel filled with boiling water.

Stir the ingredients in the container till they melt.

Add rosewater and stir further.

Store the mixture in a bottle with a large mouth, in the refrigerator, for up to a week.

Massage the mixture into your feet twice a week.

. . . .

HAIR CARE

Come winter, hair becomes dry due to inadequate moisture. This can lead to flaky dandruff and hair loss. Dryness can also lead to brittleness and inadequate sheen. There are a few quick winter care tips.

- Moisturise and nourish the scalp! Regular warm oil head massages, accompanied with the natural juices of fruits and vegetables, not only help reduce dryness but also supply vitamins and minerals to the hair.

- Coconut oil is my all time favourite hair food for winters, but sesame oil mixed with some coconut milk also brings rich rewards.

- Avoid using heated appliances as much as possible, such as blow dryers or curling irons, since they dry out the hair in winter.

- Avoid excessively hot water during hair baths. Hot water dries and damages hair! Opt for lukewarm water.

- Ensure that your hair is conditioned with a herbal conditioner to keep static at bay.

- Finally, if it is windy outside, remember to cover your hair with a scarf and protect it from the elements!

RECIPE TO NOURISH HAIR DURING WINTERS

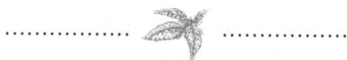

················ ················

Winter Head Massage

Ingredients

¼ cup sesame oil

1 tsp coconut milk.

Method

Mix the ingredients.

Massage the solution gently into the scalp and across the length of your hair for about 5 minutes.

Tie your hair up in a neat bun and allow the solution to soak in.

After half an hour feed your hair 'Winter Hair Food'.

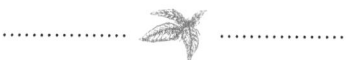

················ ················

136

Winter Hair Food

Ingredients

2 egg yolks

¼ cup papaya paste

2 tsp curd

¼ cup coconut milk

2 tsp coconut oil

4 drops ylang ylang essential oil

Method

Blend all the ingredients, except the ylang ylang, in a mixer.

Pour the paste into a glass container and add ylang ylang essential oil.

After opting for the 'Winter Head Massage' (p 136), apply the solution across the scalp and the length of your hair.

Tie your hair in a bun, and wear a shower cap to avoid staining across the nape.

Wash after 20 minutes with a mild herbal shampoo and conditioner.

Follow this ritual at least once a week for healthy locks.

················

RECIPE TO ADDRESS
DANDRUFF DURING WINTERS

Ingredients

¼ cup beetroot juice

¼ cup coconut milk

¼ cup margosa (neem) juice

1 tsp coconut oil

Method

Mix all the ingredients.

Massage this into the scalp and across the length of your hair.

Wash your hair after 20 minutes with a mild herbal shampoo and conditioner.

Follow this ritual at least once a week for healthy locks.

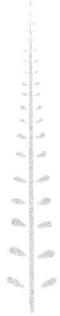

....

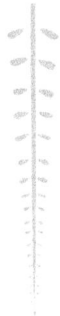

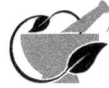

Beauty & Age
Infancy

The foetus gets all the nourishment it needs from the mother. Its skin is nurtured within the mother's body; those tufts of hair derive nutrition from the womb. Certainly, heredity plays a role, but the everyday food intake of the mother too has a direct impact on the baby's attributes. It is for this reason that a pregnant woman is urged to monitor her diet, ingest vitamins and minerals, eat fresh fruits and vegetables.

Once the baby is born, the mother has the opportunity to nurture her child the way she deems fit. I would advise all new mothers to care for the baby's skin and hair the natural way, from the time of birth.

A newborn child's skin is known to absorb every element applied to it. For this reason, it a good idea to keep the little one away from chemical soaps. It is also a good idea to embrace our grandmothers' bath recipes.

Scrub your baby with natural packs made of lentils and dry fruits. Did you know that washing your infant with a paste of green gram and oil or green gram and milk helps remove excess hair from the body? It will also make the skin soft and satiny! If your infant is very hairy, you could massage her body with egg whites before a bath. If her skin is normal, egg whites can be massaged first, and if dry, egg whites could be massaged after an oil massage. Egg whites, when used regularly, help remove superfluous hair the natural way. Interestingly, this works only during infancy, and not after!

Most infants have extremely dry skin, at times even scaly skin. In such cases, mixing green gram powder with some extra virgin olive oil, and massaging this after an oil bath, will help nourish the child's body!

Who doesn't love a massage? Babies especially love being massaged! It relaxes them, improves their circulation, and allows them to sleep soundly. Moreover, it helps psychologically too, for a mother gets to build a definite bond with her offspring! Slot a massage regimen daily or on alternate days for mother-baby time.

Massaging your little one with almond or coconut oil will help soften and nourish her skin. The choice of oil can be arrived at by massaging the baby with a particular variety of oil for a couple of days, and checking for dryness or rash patches. If there is no outbreak, you know for a fact that the oil suits the baby.

For the baby's scalp, plain coconut or almond oil will do wonders. Washing the hair with green gram powder helps keep her scalp clean and healthy.

Let me share with you the personal skin care regimen of my grandson Dhruv, who is now a year-and-a-half! When he was born, he had excellent skin, with radiant, pink feet. However, as climatic conditions changed dramatically, from a cool January to a hot and humid May, his skin colour and texture too started transforming! He developed dry and scaly skin. His mother followed a pediatrician's instructions, and doused his skin with chemical lotions.

They made no difference, and in fact, worsened the problem. Finally, at my behest, she started applying packs made of green gram and oats to his skin. His skin was very sensitive; although it lightened, it remained dry and scaly. I altered the pack. I mixed almond paste in goat's milk. It worked wonders! His skin started responding beautifully, and today it is soft like a newborn's! Since I now know that almonds suit him, I also pamper him with a pack made of saffron and dry fruits. His skin glows with appreciation!

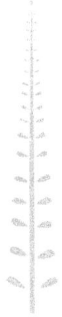

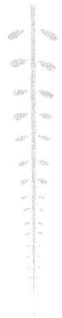

Childhood

What are your little girls made of? Sugar and spice, and all things nice. So the poem goes. Let's not take 'sugar' and 'spice' literally! For a healthy childhood and an easy transition into adolescence, sugar and spice should be consumed minimally. Have natural sugar, yes, through fruits, but keep children away from artificial sweeteners!

Children, by and large, had good skin, without even actively knowing or pursuing the fundamentals of beauty – adequate sleep, fresh air, exercise and mental calm. The fact that they had expert beauticians by their side – their mothers and grandmothers – who nurtured their skin with nature's cosmetics, meant that children were free of skin or hair ailments!

However today, the picture has changed entirely. Study stress, pollution and a diet of fast food means that children are susceptible to all the beauty problems faced by adults. Worse, mothers and grandmothers encourage remedies that revolve around bottles and tubes of chemical creams and shampoos. Chemicals may provide an easy way out of a problem, but the reprieve tends to be temporary.

Children may be lured by shampoos and cleansers with fragrances. It is however vital to train them to use natural cleansers from the very beginning. For nothing guarantees excellent skin and hair like organic food items!

BEAUTY RITUALS FOR CHILDREN

Here's a list of a few 'dos and don'ts' to preserve your little angel's skin before he or she hits puberty.

Sleep

This should be your children's greatest beauty aid. A good 8 or 9 hours of sound sleep will grant them relaxed skin and glowing eyes. Early to bed, and early to rise, makes the skin healthy, with pretty eyes!

Cleansing

Cleansing is the most important aspect of the beauty regimen. Children should avoid chemical soaps and try natural cleansers, which help the skin remain acidic. This, in turn, will help them ward off bacterial attacks. Here are a few marvellous natural cleansers for kids.

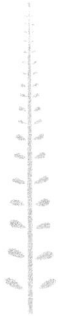

- Green gram with turmeric for those with oily skin (add buttermilk for mixing)

- Green gram with almond powder for those with dry skin (add milk for mixing)

- Oatmeal with curd for those with sensitive skin

- All these combinations could be used for the body too, but the mixing element should be milk.

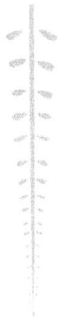

Exfoliation

Exfoliation is imperative, especially on areas like the elbows, knees, ankles and buttocks. A few natural exfoliators are.

- Dry orange peel powder with rosewater

- Wheat husk with milk

- Lemon juice with sugar granules

Moisturising

Children should moisturise their skins, but only with natural ingredients like papaya or banana mixed with honey, milk or buttermilk Attention must especially be paid to areas like the elbows, knees and ankles, which turn scaly and dark.

Apart from this, paste the following rhyme in the children's room: a dictionary on how to remain healthy!

A for apple, keeping tummy woes at bay;

B for beetroot, sending dandruff away!

C for corn, good for nerves and the brain;

D for dates, that ease all the strain!

E for eggs, with proteins for hair and body;

F for figs, which keep my bowels sturdy!

G for grapefruit, great for throat and mouth allergies;

H for honey, a storehouse of energy!

I for iodine, in spinach and beetroot;

J for jaggery, to indulge my sweet tooth!

K for kiwi; it digests the food that's doled;

L for lemon, fantastic for my cold!

M for moong sprouts, that keep me young and smart;

N for nuts, between meals and à la carte!

O for olive, massaged into my skin;

P for potatoes, with energy to win!

Q for Quaker, oats that offer skin care;

R for rice, which if brown is loved by hair!

S for soya, beans that substitute cows' milk;

T for tomato; it makes faces soft as silk!

U for U: say yes, not ifs and buts;

V for vitamins, in green veggies, fruits and nuts!

W for wheat germ, making rotis doubly yummy;

X is an exit, no to junk food that hurts tummies!

Y for yoghurt, which cleanses face and hair;

Z for zeal: I must follow this with care!

FACE CARE

Apart from a regular routine of cleansing-exfoliating-moisturising, when your children are inching towards adolescence, it is especially important to follow a more careful skin care regime. At this point, the skin could become excessively oily or even burst into a few eruptions. A simple pack could help prevent and curtail this.

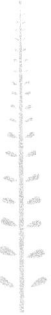

RECIPE TO ADDRESS OILY SKIN

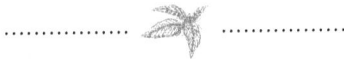

Child-Friendly Oily Skin Pack

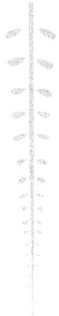

Ingredients

2 slices cucumber

8-9 marigold petals

5-6 holy basil (tulsi) leaves

Method

Grind these ingredients together to form a paste.

Apply this twice daily across the face and neck.

Wash off after 5 minutes with lukewarm water.

Apply daily till the condition improves.

BODY CARE

Some children hate having a daily bath, but it is important to get them into the habit. Others may not enjoy long-winded beauty rituals with packs and potions. In such cases, an oatmeal bath would do the trick. This not only softens the skin but also provides it with natural vitamins.

RECIPE FOR A WEEKLY BATH

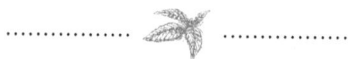

Child-Friendly Oatmeal Bath

Ingredients

1 cup oatmeal powder

1 tsp sandalwood powder

5-6 rose petals, powdered

1 cup thick milk

3 tsp lentil powder (optional)

5-6 margosa (neem) leaves, powdered (optional)

Method

Take a single pair of socks, and pour the oatmeal and sandalwood powders into them.

Now add the crushed rose petals.

You could add the lentil powder and margosa leaves too.

Soak the socks in the cup of milk for 20 minutes.

Rub the socks all over your child's body, letting the mixture seep out gently.

Bathe your child with the milk that is left.

Now wash him or her with lukewarm water.

Follow this once a week, to soften scaly and dry skin! Your child will enjoy the ritual, and won't feel like its a porridge bath!

RECIPE TO SCRUB THE BODY

.... 🌿 ....

Child-Friendly Soap-Free Body Scrub

Ingredients

½ cup green gram powder

½ cup oatmeal powder

½ cup turmeric powder

2 tsp margosa (neem) powder

1 cup milk

Method

Place all the ingredients, except the milk, in a huge stainless steel sieve and filter. The sieve helps remove poorly ground pieces and allows the powders to mix well.

Store this mixture in a glass container in a fridge.

While having a bath, blend the mixture with milk, and apply it evenly across the body.

Wash off after 5 minutes with lukewarm water.

Apply once a week, for glowing, exfoliated skin!

147

....

RECIPE TO ADDRESS TANNING

....

Children love playing in the sun, or swimming. Of course, the immediate consequence of this is that they get tanned! Kitchen ingredients can come to the rescue!

Child-Friendly Tan Remover

Ingredients

1 cup split red lentils (masoor dal), washed, dried and powdered

½ tsp turmeric powder

2 tsp red sandalwood paste

2 cups milk

Method

Mix the split red lentils, turmeric powder and sandalwood paste, with half a cup of milk, to get a pack.

Apply this across the face, neck, hands and legs.

Wash off with the remaining milk and then water after 5 minutes.

Apply regularly so the skin lightens.

HANDS AND FEET CARE

As vital as it is to care for a child's skin, it is equally important to attend to the nails. If they're nursed at an early stage, chances are, the nails will be smooth and healthy tomorrow!

To prevent a case of chipped nails, massage a little olive or almond oil into the nails at night. To make them even stronger, soak them once a month in warm water to which 2 dashes of gelatine are added.

Encourage your children to consume oats, brown rice, sprouts, fruits, fresh vegetables and dry fruits. If they resist, try making food look colourful and appealing, so they eat fresh and healthy!

HAIR CARE

Let's maintain the tresses of our children the natural way!

If you wish to promote hair growth, start tending to the locks of your little girl or boy by the time she or he is 6. Massaging coconut oil with some coconut milk helps.

Apart from this, here are some quick and easy recipes!

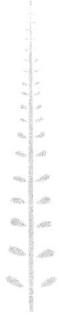

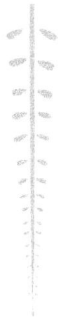

RECIPE FOR A HAIR CLEANSER

....

Child-Friendly Hair Bath

Ingredients

¼ cup fenugreek (methi) seeds

5-6 hibiscus petals

5-6 margosa (neem) leaves

Method

Soak the fenugreek seeds in water.

The next day, grind them with the hibiscus petals and margosa leaves.

Sieve the ground mixture.

Add a little water to the filtered mixture, to get a smooth paste.

Massage this into the scalp and hair.

After letting it soak in for half an hour, use a mild herbal shampoo and conditioner.

Follow this once a week; the mixture will promote hair growth, and control dandruff and premature greying.

Note: You could also blend the sieved mixture with milk, egg white and/or honey.

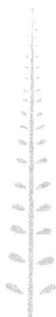

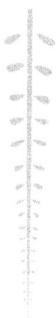

....

RECIPE TO ADDRESS LIGHT COLOURED HAIR

Child-Friendly Hair Darkener

Ingredients

6 tsp coconut oil

1 tsp curry leaf juice

1 tsp coconut milk

Method

Mix the ingredients.

Massage this into the scalp and across the length of your child's hair.

Let this soak in for an hour.

Wash off with a mild herbal shampoo and conditioner.

Follow this once a week for beautiful dark hair.

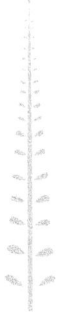

151

RECIPE TO ADDRESS DANDRUFF

Child-Friendly Dandruff Fighter

Ingredients

2 tsp margosa (neem) juice

2 tsp beetroot juice

6 tsp coconut oil

Method

Mix the ingredients.

Massage this into the scalp and across the length of your child's hair.

Let this soak in for an hour.

Now wash off with a mild herbal shampoo and conditioner.

Follow this once a week for dandruff-free hair.

RECIPE TO ADDRESS LICE

Your children are off to school! How exciting! But then, they come back home with guests on their hair – mighty lice, sucking in nutrition from their scalp.

Lice infestation not only deprives the scalp of nourishment, but also causes excessive hair loss, itchiness, and a lot of embarrassment! Lice multiply very fast. Worse, they can pass from your child to you, which is double trouble!

It's therefore vital to take care of your children's hair from the very first school day. In case they bring home lice however, here is a natural remedy.

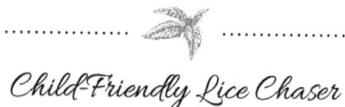

....

Child-Friendly Lice Chaser

Ingredients

4 tsp coconut oil, warmed

2 tsp margosa (neem) oil

4 tsp margosa (neem) juice

Method

Massage the warm coconut oil and margosa oil into the scalp and across the length of your child's hair.

Then massage some margosa juice into the scalp.

Tie the hair with a thin muslin cloth tightly for 5 minutes.

Then open out the hair, and using a fine toothed lice comb, run through the tresses to remove all lice.

Wash the hair with a margosa based shampoo and conditioner.

Once again, tie the hair with a thin muslin cloth, and wipe it dry gently.

Now, a second time around, comb the hair to remove lice.

To remove all nits, ensure that your little one's scalp is clean.

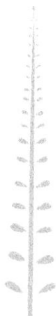

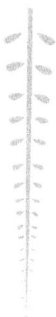

....

Adolescence

Adolescents tend to get especially embarrassed about their appearance. They worry over zits, and become weight conscious. Tanning makes them ill at ease, and bad hair days drive them to tears.

Perhaps the best advice one can give teens is this: Follow a nutritious diet chart. In other words, adolescents must stay away from junk food. They should also not cut down on sensible fare, such as fresh and dry fruits, required for growth and energy. Emphasizing this is critical since anorexia can sneak up on teens, depriving their body of mineral rich fodder.

The hair quality of adolescents is influenced by their food patterns. Therefore, they should eat vegetables (salads), brown rice and oats for vitamin B; oily fish and flax seeds for omega-3 fatty acids; shellfish and pumpkin seeds for zinc; dates, raisins and prunes for iron; low fat dairy products for calcium; and Brazil nuts for selenium. Olive and safflower oil offer polysaturates; avocados, sunflower oil and peanut butter (without salt) are rich in vitamin E.

Apples, apricots, guava, melons, grapes, strawberries, kiwi, oranges and lemons are all good for the skin. Every adolescent's best friend should be the colour green. They should include it in their everyday menu, even if it is in the form of simple coriander. These vegetables come with reserves of beta-carotene, which in turn supplies vitamin A, essential for healthy skin and clear eyes. The green in

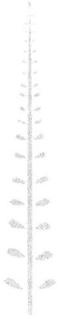

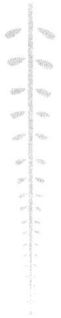

fresh vegetables also offers chlorophyll, which keeps the skin clear, and has nourishing and antiseptic properties.

Without doubt, liquids, including pure water, tender coconut and fresh fruit and vegetable juices, make the skin young and healthy. A simple drink made from cucumbers, carrots, beetroot and a single Indian gooseberry, with a few dashes of lime, can make the complexion glow.

ACNE

The biggest bugbear for adolescents is the pimple that erupts without warning! One boil can make them run for cover. The truth is youngsters look good, even if they have a zit or two. They need to be confident in themselves, and know that a few pimples do not make them unattractive. Once they develop such self confidence, and stop being paranoid, one can begin addressing the skin problem, and correct or reduce the causes responsible for it.

There are many factors that encourage acne assaults: stress, lack of sleep, poor hygiene, low-grade cosmetics, constipation, heredity, dandruff and improper diet. Once these causes are addressed, the skin clears up.

A simple suggestion for all teens: Do not ever play with or burst a pimple or a boil, for you could scar yourself; these marks can stay for a very long time. Another suggestion: Avoid shellfish, prawns, cashewnuts, iodised salt, coffee, tea and sugar; steer clear of junk food.

Besides this, natural packs are recommended. If organic packs have been applied from childhood, teenage skin and hair ailments will be few and far between. However, for those of us who have missed such childhood care, pampering can begin in the teens as well! Dip into nature's reserves if an adolescent's hormones are on a roller coaster. Include fruits and salads not only in the diet, but in everyday face packs too.

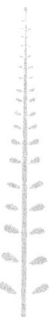

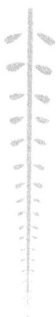

RECIPES TO ADDRESS TEENAGE ACNE

Note: In the remedies that follow, I have recommended washing the face with buttermilk. This is to create an acid mantle which can prevent bacterial attacks.

....

Mint-Margosa Teenage Acne Buster

Ingredients

25 mint leaves

12 margosa (neem) leaves

¼ cucumber

1 tsp honey

¼ cup buttermilk or cucumber juice

Method

Grind the above ingredients, except the buttermilk or cucumber juice, to get a paste.

Apply twice daily across the face and neck.

After 5 minutes, wash off with some buttermilk or cucumber juice and then water.

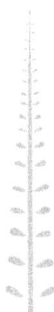

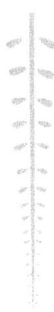

....

Sandalwood Turmeric Teenage Acne Buster

Ingredients

1 tsp sandalwood paste

¼ tsp wild turmeric paste

1 tsp honey

¼ tsp rose petal powder

¼ cup buttermilk

Method

Mix all the ingredients, except the buttermilk, to get a smooth paste.

Apply this gently across the face and neck.

Wash off after 5 minutes with some buttermilk and then plain cold water.

Follow this daily for results.

....

COLOURED HAIR

A teenager is always but always tempted to experiment with his/her hair. Teens find past hairstyles boring, and original hair colour uninteresting. They straighten, perm, dye, and streak their locks for novelty, to keep up with trends, and to stand out among peers.

However, chemical tampering can damage the hair's structure, thereby causing it to thin, break and fall.

Ideally, teenagers should avoid exposing their hair to chemicals. But as we know, experimenting and being an adolescent go hand in hand. Therefore, what teens can do is address all issues that surround coloured hair the natural way!

RECIPE TO ADDRESS COLOURED HAIR

················ ················

Papaya Damaged Hair Saviour

Ingredients

1 cup papaya paste

1 cup coconut milk

1 cup aloe vera pulp

½ cup olive oil

2 dashes ylang ylang oil

Method

Blend all the ingredients, except the ylang ylang oil, in a glass container.

Now add ylang ylang oil.

Apply the mixed potion to the scalp and hair.

After 20 minutes, use a herbal shampoo and a conditioner like aloe vera gel.

Follow this ritual before every hair wash for results.

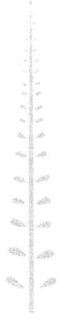

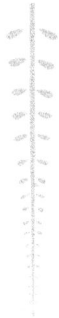

157

RECIPE TO FOSTER HAIR GROWTH

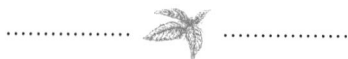

.... 🌿 ....

Coconut-Egg Hair Growth Potion

Ingredients

½ cup olive oil

½ cup coconut milk

2 eggs

½ cup extra virgin coconut oil

½ cup fenugreek (methi) seed juice

2 dashes rosemary oil

Method

Massage warm olive oil across the scalp and hair for 5 minutes.

Now mix the remaining ingredients in a glass container, adding the rosemary oil at the end.

Apply the potion across the scalp and hair.

After 20 minutes, use a herbal shampoo and a conditioner.

Follow this ritual before every hair wash for results.

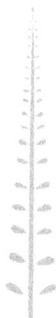

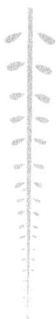

....

The Prime of Life

Every age marks a beautiful stage in life. Ageing signifies maturity. And maturity means that your life is in full bloom.

Sadly, a lot of us fear ageing. We look at ourselves in the mirror, spot our first grey hair or a wrinkle, and get alarmed. We rush to cosmetic surgeons, assuming they will rid us of this menace! The truth is, there is no magic potion to make time stand still. Despite the claims of the cosmetic industry – that it can reverse ageing through Botox, fillers, peels and surgeries – growing old is inevitable, and needs to be accepted gracefully.

Let me make my point clear: Ageing is definite. While it can't be stalled, it can be slowed down.

A lot of us instinctively rush to cosmetic surgeons to slow down ageing. It can't be denied that the cosmetic industry has made giant leaps in the fields of skin grafting and plastic surgery. But these processes are foreign, alien to the body's natural state. Therefore, while the early results offered by these chemicals are amazing, new problems or old ones erupt and recur shortly after opting for these miracle cures.

Instead of hitting the panic button, rushing for quick-fix cosmetic procedures to reverse ageing, and risking serious side effects, maybe we could try making simple changes in our lifestyle and diet to control ageing naturally. This will not only help us look youthful but also keep us fit and increase longevity.

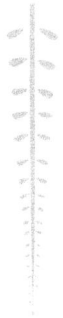

Scientific studies reveal that on an average our bodies are at their youthful peak at 25; signs of ageing surface at 30. However, we all age at different rates. Genetic factors, gender, ethnicity, environmental influences, levels of sun exposure and lifestyle choices like smoking, drinking and nutrition are factors that predetermine ageing.

The process of controlling ageing should start right from the time when age isn't even a concern – right after puberty. It may be difficult to restore youth after age has ravaged the body. So why not start young?

How Does One Slow Down Ageing?

Exercise
Regular exercise will keep you in shape, improve posture, enhance energy levels, keep joints supple, strengthen muscles and increase blood circulation. Your skin therefore will glow with health.

Exercise also helps feed the brain with oxygen; therefore, you stay alert even as you grow older.

It is important to choose the exercise that suits you after consulting a doctor. As you age, it's wise to reduce the intensity of your working-out regime, and opt for moderate exercises like walking, jogging, yoga, swimming or golf, none of which get you out of breath and sweaty.

A Healthy Diet
A healthy diet should include carbohydrates, proteins, fats, vitamins and minerals in the right proportion to provide the body with energy and all the nutrients it needs for growth and repair.

As we grow older we need fewer calories to sustain us. But we still need as many vitamins and minerals as we've always had. Sometimes nutritional supplements may help.

Vitamin A helps remove age spots. Biotin, choline and folic acid prevent the greying of hair. Vitamin C can arrest wrinkles. Drink at least 8 glasses of water a day to prevent the skin from looking dull and dry, flush out toxins from the body, prevent constipation and keep the bowels healthy. Quit smoking and drinking.

Regular Health Checkups
Visit the doctor regularly to check for symptoms of age-related ailments like heart and circulatory diseases, diabetes, back pain, arthritis, osteoporosis and cancer. Being in the pink of health will make you look your youthful best.

Skin Care
The outer covering and the largest organ of the body, the skin, is the very first organ to show signs of ageing. The skin loses elasticity, gets thinner and dries up as we grow old. Sun contact, smoking, alcohol consumption, stress, inadequate sleep, prolonged periods of illness, exposure to pollution and chemicals, and a poor diet can cause wrinkles early. Overusing soap, and excessive steaming and bleaching may further dry up the skin.

Face massages with essential oils, acupressure and facial exercises may help to prevent wrinkles.

Hair Care
Hard water, harsh chemicals, excessive shampooing, driers and rollers may hasten the greying of hair.

On the other hand, consuming or applying Indian gooseberries, curry leaves, fenugreek seeds and coconut milk will naturally darken your mane. Scalp massages with rosemary oil in a base of almond, olive or jojoba oil increase blood circulation, bringing nutrients and oxygen to hair follicles. Lavender or thyme oil stimulate hair growth. Also, a diet rich in minerals and vitamins can prevent hair loss.

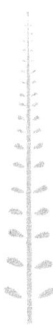

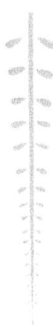

Nail Care

Brittle nails are caused by hard water or a deficiency in vitamins and minerals. White spots on the nails suggest a zinc or vitamin B deficiency. Lack of iron leads to pale, flat, thin and dry nails.

For healthy and strong nails, have a diet rich in sulphur, iron, zinc, calcium and vitamins. Wear rubber gloves while cleaning or washing. Practise hand and finger exercises regularly.

Dental Care

Common dental problems affecting senior citizens include tooth decay, gum disease, fractures and normal wearing away of the enamel.

Avoid extracting natural teeth unless absolutely necessary as they help anchor artificial teeth.

Vitamin D helps absorb calcium and keep teeth healthy. Follow good oral hygiene by regular brushing, flossing and gum massages.

Eye Care

Rest ensures that your eyes aren't strained or tired.

When your eyes get weary, close them and press your eyelids very gently with your palms. While reading, choose a relaxing place with comfortable light. Go for regular eye checkups for sight problems, macular degeneration, glaucoma and cataracts. Finally, have a diet rich in vitamin A.

Being Young at Heart

Though society may categorise your years numerically, real age is linked to your mind. If you think young, you'll look young. If you have a happy and peaceful mind, the lines of stress won't show on you. Therefore you'll look much younger.

Going Natural

Nature holds the elixir of youth. Remember to dip into the world's many organic treasures to remain forever young.

RECIPES TO CONTROL AGEING

Use any of these packs on a daily basis for youthful, glowing skin.

....

Aroma Fruit Pack

Ingredients

4 tsp papaya paste

4 tsp avacado paste

1 tsp almond oil

1 dash ylang ylang essential oil

Method

Mix all of the ingredients in a glass bowl.

Massage this paste across the face and neck.

After 5-10 minutes, wash off with cold water.

....

Honey Fruit Pack

Ingredients

2 egg yolks

2 tsp honey

4 tsp almond powder

1 dash ylang ylang essential oil

Method

Beat the egg yolks in a glass container with honey, almond powder and the ylang ylang essential oil.

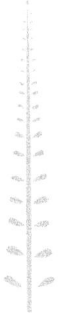

Massage this viscous paste across the face and neck in quick, upward strokes.

After 5-10 minutes, wash off with cold water and then alternate by splashing cold and hot water a few times.

....

Dry Fruit Pack

Ingredients

4 tsp coconut milk

10-12 almonds

2 tsp almond oil

1 tsp honey

Method

Soak the almonds overnight. Now peel them and grind them into a paste.

Mix the almond paste with the coconut milk, almond oil and honey.

Massage this pack across the face and neck.

Wash off with lukewarm water after 5-10 minutes.

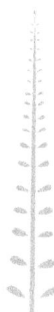

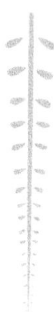

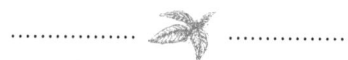

Fruit-o-licious

Ingredients

6 strawberries

½ banana

2 tsp almond oil

2 tsp oatmeal powder

½ cup milk

Method

Boil the strawberries for 2 minutes.

Now grind them with banana, almond oil and oatmeal powder, to get a paste.

Apply a thick coat of the paste across the face and neck for about 5-10 minutes.

Wash off the pack with some milk and then rinse with water.

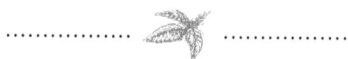

Aloe Fruit Pack

Ingredients

4 tsps orange juice

4 tsps + ¼ cup cucumber juice

2 tsp green gram powder

2 tsp aloe vera pulp

1 dash apple cider vinegar

Method

Mix the orange juice, green gram powder, and aloe vera pulp, with 4 teaspoons of cucumber juice, to get a paste.

Apply this across the face and neck.

Now mix apple cider vinegar with the remaining half cup of cucumber juice.

When the pack on the face and neck feels semi-dry, wash off with the cucumber juice and apple cider vinegar mixture.

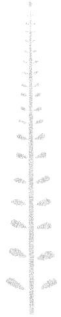

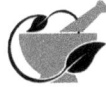

Beauty & the Man

Introduction

Beauty is no longer chiefly a 'female' concern. Today, men are equally conscious of their looks.

This is just as well, since all men need to tend to their skin and hair. If they don't bother about hygiene, they could very well end up with boils and pimples and dandruff. Apart from this, tanning, sunburn, premature greying, and hair fall are just a few problems that don't spare men!

SKIN CARE

There are natural recipes that specifically attend to problems faced by men, and address male skin. However it is entirely safe for men to dip into the packs listed under the general skin and hair care segments as well. Therefore, if fighting acne or rosacea, for instance, the recipes listed under those sections can be used by everyone, irrespective of gender.

Skin Softening

Little boys have delicate skin. As they inch towards their torrid teens, their skin starts thickening. The skin of men in general is thicker than that of women; hence the average man needs more exfoliation than women.

Here is a pack that works wonders, making male skin baby soft.

RECIPE TO SOFTEN MALE SKIN

....

Papaya-Almond Skin Softener

Ingredients

½ cup papaya paste

4 tsp almond powder

¼ cup milk

Method

Mix the ingredients to form a paste.

Apply this across the face and neck.

After 5 minutes, wash off with cool water.

Apply daily for smooth, soft skin.

....

Post-Shaving Care

A common male concern is shaving, which can make skin rough and dry. All men should opt for a 100 per cent natural aftershave lotion to combat this problem.

RECIPE FOR AN AFTERSHAVE LOTION

....

The All Natural Aftershave Lotion

Ingredients

4 tsp aloe vera juice

4 tsp cucumber juice

2 dashes tea tree oil

Method

Mix all the ingredients together.

Splash the liquid across the face after a shave.

Then splash cold water.

Follow this ritual after every shave for smooth skin.

....

Tanning

Men's bodies face fewer hormonal ups and downs; as a result men are less likely to develop problems like pigmentation. Of course, if they have flawed genes, or outdoor jobs, pigmentation is likely to be a problem for the best of men!

Those men who spend long hours outdoors should take practical care. They should carry glares and an umbrella, and wear full-length clothes. Apart from this, there are packs that can address tanning.

RECIPE TO ADDRESS TANNING

Tan Fighter for Men

Ingredients	Method
2 tsp red lentils (masoor dal) powder	Mix the ingredients to form a smooth paste.
3 tsp milk	Apply this paste across the face and the neck.
2 dashes lime	After 5 minutes, wash off with cold water.
	Apply regularly after a day outdoors.

HANDS AND FEET CARE

While attending to their facial skin and hair, men should remember to look after their hands and feet too. In general, they should wear comfortable shoes, and regularly moisturise their hands.

Unkempt nails or dry hands are unbecoming and can make one lose confidence. A daily 2-minute hand and foot care ritual can do wonders to tackle this problem.

For clean hands and feet, dip your feet for about 15 minutes in a tub filled with warm water to which margosa (neem) leaves, slices of lime and a few drops of essential oils like lavender, sage or pine oil are added.

Happy hands and feet make happy men.

HAIR CARE

Premature Greying

A problem faced by several men is premature greying.

Ideally, if there are only a few strands of grey, natural henna should be used. This not only hides the streaks of white, but also keeps hair healthy and strong.

Those who grey early and in profusion have no option but to colour their hair. Care should be taken to use natural products regularly to balance the side effects of chemical colouring.

Dandruff

Men with dandruff tend to get especially embarrassed since it appears in patches on their black suits and dark sweaters.

There are a few simple steps that can be followed by all men to avoid being 'snowed under'. For one, they can stay away from very hot water while washing their hair, and steer clear of hair dryers. They should use lukewarm water instead and allow their hair to dry naturally. Secondly, men should keep time aside to oil and massage their scalp and hair once a week.

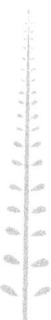

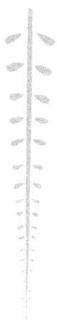

RECIPE TO ADDRESS DANDRUFF

.... 🌿 ....

Anti-Dandruff Beetroot Cure

Ingredient

½ beetroot, grated

½ cup apple cider vinegar

Method

Squeeze out the juice from the beetroot.

Apply this thrice a week to the scalp.

After 10 minutes, wash off with plain water mixed with apple cider vinegar.

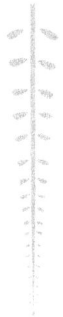

....

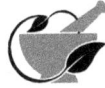

Beauty & Weddings
Introduction

From time immemorial, weddings in India have been associated with celebration, holy rites, feasts and music. While the ceremony per se may vary from culture to culture, across the east, west, north and south, each ritual is linked with fulfilment and joy.

The bride has always been the centre of care and pampering during weddings. From the days of yore, brides have been doused in natural ingredients, so their skin and hair get cleansed, moisturised and nourished. It's not unusual for a bride's body to be smeared with turmeric. In some cultures, brides are encouraged to have a bath in a tub of water filled with rose petals, margosa or neem leaves and cut lime pieces. Other cultures promote the use of aromatic oils; they believe scrubbing the bride's body with natural fragrances will keep evil spirits at bay! Still others believe that the use of face packs made of wild turmeric, sandalwood, saffron and rosewater grant the bride's face allure and sheen, and hair packs of curry and margosa leaves, hibiscus and soap nut grant the tresses lustre.

I'd like to emphasise a point here. While a lot of marriage and pre-marriage beauty rituals aim to make the bride look her radiant best, they aren't meant to make her 'fair'. Colour doesn't symbolise beauty, healthy skin and hair does. And the packs and potions that are applied merely rid the skin of blemishes, tanning and signs of age.

For years, beauty was divorced from masculinity, and little attention was paid to the attractiveness of the groom. Thankfully, a lot of that has changed with time, and these days, grooms visit parlours to get facials, clean their nails and tend to their hair.

Today, thanks to the Hindi and South Indian film industries and television soaps, marriages have become enormously commercial, in terms of decor, lights, music, food and dress codes. We have entered an era of theme weddings. We have also entered an era where brides and grooms spend months before the actual wedding beautifying themselves. I have a single recommendation to make: Pamper the skin and hair with natural products instead of chemical ingredients.

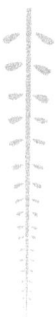

Post-Engagement

In most Indian cultures, the magni, nichayathartham, engagement or betrothal precedes a wedding. It is the first sign of a lifelong commitment. In most cases, the gap between the engagement and the wedding is not too long, and anywhere between 3 and 6 months.

This gives the couple just about enough time to start taking care of themselves. Even while attending to multiple things – the booking of venues, the printing of invites, shopping and catering – brides and grooms have a tiny window to attend to their beauty.

Pre-bridal or groom skin and hair care ideally should start at least 3 to 6 months in advance. You may well ask, why does one need all this time?

There are a few key reasons. With regards to skin care, one needs to arrive at the perfect set of ingredients and the ideal pack for an individual's skin type. In case of an allergic outbreak, one needs to have a little time to undo the problem.

With regards to the hair, results can be seen only after 2 or 3 months. Moreover, since the hair will be exposed to various styling procedures on the wedding day, including heat application and chemical sprays, it needs a lot of nourishment and strengthening prior.

Here are some pre-bridal/groom recipes for the skin and hair, which with a little effort can be followed at home twice a week for at least a month.

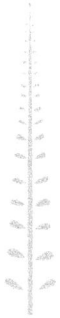

SKIN CARE

Brides- and grooms-to-be can use a range of cleansers to get glowing skin.

RECIPE FOR OILY SKIN

Tomato-Cucumber Cleanser

Ingredients	Method
½ tomato	Grind the ingredients to get a paste.
½ cucumber	
	Apply this across the face and neck if you have oily skin.
	After 5 minutes, wash off with lukewarm water.

176

RECIPE FOR ACNE-PRONE SKIN

Margosa-Cucumber Cleanser

Ingredients	Method
¼ cup cucumber juice	Mix the ingredients to get a paste.
1 tsp margosa (neem) paste	
	Apply this twice a day across the face and neck if acne-prone.
	After 5 minutes, wash off with lukewarm water.

RECIPE FOR DRY SKIN

.... 🌿 ....

Almond-Curd Cleanser

Ingredients

10 almonds

¼ cup curd

Method

Grind the almonds to get a powder.

Now mix this with curd, till you get a paste.

Apply this across the face and neck if you have very dry skin.

After 5 minutes, wash off with lukewarm water.

....

RECIPE TO ADDRESS TANNED BACKS

While attending to their faces, brides- and grooms-to-be often neglect their backs. Make sure to cleanse this part of the body. A paste of almond, oats and honey is a sure way of brightening it.

Apply from this, here is an excellent scrub.

.... 🌿 ....

Oatmeal-Turmeric Paste

Ingredients

½ cup oatmeal flour

1 tsp turmeric powder

4 tsp coconut milk

Method

Mix all the ingredients to get a paste.

Apply this across the back.

The hands and feet are equally important and these packs can be applied liberally on them too.

Wash off after 5-10 minutes with lukewarm water.

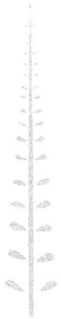

....

HAIR CARE

Brides- and grooms-to-be need to invest time in strengthening their hair. This is to prevent a case of damaged hair after the wedding.

RECIPE TO STRENGTHEN AND ADD VOLUME TO THE HAIR

Note: The quantities of the ingredients can be proportionately increased, if the hair is thick and long.

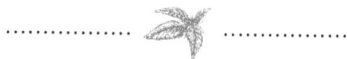

....

Fenugreek Hair Repairer

Ingredients

¼ cup fenugreek (methi) juice

¼ cup coconut milk

¼ cup papaya paste

½ cup coconut oil, warmed

Method

Massage warm coconut oil into the scalp for 5 minutes.

Now mix the fenugreek juice, papaya paste and coconut milk together.

Massage this into the scalp for 5 minutes.

Wash the mixture off after 20 minutes with a mild herbal shampoo and conditioner.

Follow this at least once a week for strong, nourished hair.

....

The Month Before the Wedding

The month before the wedding is an exciting period. However, given the amount that needs to be attended to, late nights become frequent, missed meals become regular affairs, and stress is an everyday emotion.

For some, the idea of marriage itself creates anxiety, and stokes fears and apprehensions. This, in turn, causes sleepless nights, which can lead to dark circles, pimples, dandruff and dull skin. Those who trousseau shop in the afternoons can face the additional problem of tanning and sunburn.

In the month before the wedding, make a conscious effort to schedule your day in terms of meals, exercises and rest, so your body maintains a healthy equilibrium. Follow a diet which includes whole grains and nuts, seasonal fruits and vegetables, hot soups and lots of water.

Professionals should try being organised, so they can wind up work before the wedding.

Equally, try investing time in natural beauty procedures instead of chemical ones. Bleaching and peels may offer temporary results, but they come with harmful side effects and cause long term skin damage.

In the 5 weeks before the wedding, brides and grooms should take a regular bath with a paste made of green gram, turmeric, margosa leaves, almond oil and milk. This will remove all grime and keep the skin soft and polished.

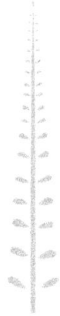

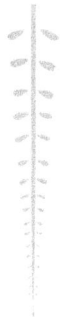

They should also nurture their face daily with a fruit pack; the vitamins will lend a glow to the skin.

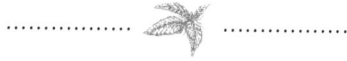

....

Bride-n-Groom Fruit Pack

Ingredients

¼ orange, peeled and deseeded

¼ carrot

¼ cucumber

1 tsp extra virgin coconut oil

Method

Extract the juice of the orange, carrot and cucumber to fill half a cup.

Add the extra virgin coconut oil. (Note: Those with oily skin need not use oil.)

Apply the mixture across the face and neck repeatedly till you have used it all up.

After 10 minutes, splash cold water twice or thrice across the face and neck.

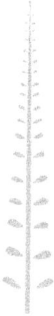

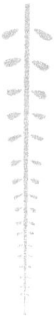

The Wedding

HALDI KI RASAM

The wedding day is drawing close! One of the most important functions across several communities a day before the wedding is 'haldi ki rasam', or the turmeric bath – a must for both the bride and the groom. This is often observed before the mehendi, so that the colour of the paste doesn't fade.

The bride or the groom is made to sit on a small stool. Amidst fun and frolic, song and dance, the relatives and friends smear turmeric paste on the body of the couple. This leads to bright and glowing skin, and improved tone and texture, all appropriate for a wedding! Sometimes, turmeric is blended with sandalwood and used as a scrub to enhance the quality of the skin.

However, it is important to remember that the quality of the ingredients is of paramount importance. Today's adulterated, readymade spices can do more harm than good. Ensure that the spices are either homemade or sourced from entirely reliable places. Equally, do bear in mind that turmeric may not suit everyone; some are allergic to it. Today's brides and grooms therefore should try a patch test at least some weeks before the wedding to check the ingredient's suitability. If allergic to turmeric, one could make a facial pack to suit the skin, and merely add a single teaspoon of turmeric for the sake of following an old ritual.

Ideally, one should try mixing sandalwood and other herbs to avoid a case of skin over-sensitivity. Those with dry skin could discover that turmeric irritates and further dehydrates their bodies. Hence mixing it with little buttermilk and some oil will deliver results.

I have created some simple recipes that will enhance skin tone. These could be used as a part of the haldi ki rasam ritual.

RECIPE FOR NORMAL SKIN

.... 🌿 ....

Red Lentils Rite

Ingredients

3 tsp red lentils (masoor dal), soaked overnight

4 almonds, soaked overnight and peeled

2 tsp coconut milk + 1 cup coconut milk

1 tsp turmeric paste

Method

Mix all the above ingredients, except the full cup of coconut milk, to get a paste.

Apply this across the face and the neck for 5 minutes.

After 5-10 minutes, wash off with the full cup of coconut milk, and then water.

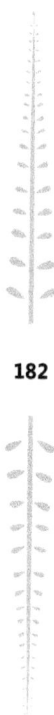

....

RECIPE FOR DRY SKIN

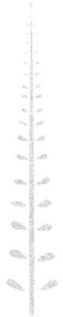

Almonds-Orange Rite

Ingredients

4 almonds

4 tsp orange juice

4 tsp cucumber juice

2 tsp almond oil

1 tsp turmeric paste

1 cup milk

Method

Mix all the above ingredients, except the milk, to get a paste.

Apply this across the face and neck.

After 5-10 minutes, wash with milk, and then water.

RECIPE FOR OILY / ACNE-PRONE SKIN

Turmeric-Holy Basil Rite

Ingredients

1 tsp turmeric paste

10 holy basil (tulsi) leaves

10 mint leaves

½ cucumber

2 tsp green gram powder

Method

Grind all the ingredients together to get a smooth paste.

Apply across the face and neck.

After 5-10 minutes, wash off with lukewarm water.

SPECIAL CARE FOR THE MONSOON BRIDE AND GROOM

Whatever the season, the bride and the groom are expected to look their best. This becomes an especial challenge during the monsoons.

Rain woes can be huge in number. The uneven distribution of moisture can lead to dull, unhealthy skin. This problem can be addressed by choosing a quick-fix facial, appropriate to the skin type, from the ones listed in the book.

Perhaps the biggest concern in the rainy season is that hair becomes limp and lifeless! How can this issue be addressed? Nature has the answer.

RECIPE TO ADDRESS LIMP HAIR

The Wedding Bad Hair Day Cure

Ingredients

1 egg, beaten well

1 egg white

4 tsp henna powder

½ cup papaya paste

4 drops rosemary oil

Method

Mix all the ingredients, except the rosemary oil, in a blender.

Pour them into a glass bowl.

Now add the rosemary oil.

Those with extremely dry hair could mix in 2 tsp curd and 2 tsp olive oil too.

Apply the paste all over scalp and hair, making segments, and tie or pin this up.

After 20 minutes, wash off with a mild herbal shampoo and conditioner.

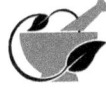

Case Studies
& Testimonials

Dr Roopa Shetty
Franchise Owner, Nirmal Herbal

I have always been a believer in natural, freshly ground products, and think they should be used in shampoos, conditioners, hair packs, and face packs.

Around 12 years ago, I had got my hair straightened with strong chemicals. A month or two after, I started experiencing severe hair loss. I met Dr Shetty, and followed an 'all natural' regimen. I started soaking fenugreek seeds at night along with curry leaves, grinding these into a paste, and applying the juice on the scalp. This treatment started giving me great results, controlled hair fall, and within few weeks fresh growth of hair was visible! All this further assured me of the benefits of natural ingredients, when used in beauty products.

Divya Padmanabhan
Manager: Business Development, Times of India (Corporate)

My first interaction with Dr Shetty was in the year 2007. I was paranoid about hair fall, had bad hair days and acne breakouts all over the face. Doctor (as I fondly address her) reassured me that everything would be fine if I followed a natural regimen. I learnt that simple kitchen ingredients could make all the difference to your overall wellbeing and beauty.

First, the acne breakouts were triggered by dandruff and flakes on the scalp, which needed to be addressed. So the suggested plan was diet modification (internal) and also external care of hair.

My diet was modified to include lots of fresh vegetables and fruits, along with antioxidants (which meant having either green tea or orange juice every day). My diet also came to include a lot of cucumber and carrot before meals, followed by a normal home cooked lunch or dinner. On Doctor's advice, I opted for bajra or jowar rotis (instead of wheat rotis), and brown rice (instead of white rice).

External care included applying a hair paste of papaya and curd, massaging the scalp with Indian gooseberry and fenugreek juice, and then washing the hair with a hibiscus shampoo once a week. Coconut milk massages, and egg and yoghurt packs also helped stimulate hair follicles.

Within 3 months, my hair fall stopped completely and I could also see visible hair growth. The texture of my hair improved drastically and my hair also increased in length.

Along with hair care, Doctor had also suggested a skin care regime, which would include washing my face with curd every time it was exposed to the sun. Once a week, I would apply orange and carrot juice as it helped tone the skin. I also got facials done with saffron, dry fruits and milk. This granted a visible glow to my face.

After years of going natural, I completely believe in this approach intellectually. It has an impressive spiritual lineage too!

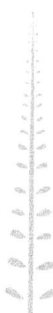

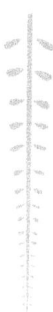

Sheena Saji
Former General Manager, DNA

Nature does not hurry, yet everything is accomplished. So Lao Tzu said rather aptly. All my life, I have been fond of everything that is natural and in the purest form. This is reflected in everything I do – from my choice of food to my preferences for interior design.

It's nice to embrace the natural beauty within you. This thought was emphasised by Dr Nirmala Shetty. She made me realise the benefits of being in sync with nature!

My beauty regimen used to be very simple – sunscreen and moisturising, eyeliner and a dash of lipstick. My skin was very sensitive, so I never experimented. No facial, no bleaching, no foundation – in short nothing beyond a regular face wash.

For the past 18 years though, I have been consulting Dr Shetty, and doing regular natural facial clean ups, hair treatment and pedicures. I also try to get at least 8 hours of sleep, drink a lot of water and exercise. I sincerely feel that beauty largely comes from within. You are what you eat!

Prabha Narayanan
Chief Secretarial Assistant

One day, Dr Shetty asked me why I had developed pimples over my face and a large colony of pimples on my forehead. I explained that I have irregular periods. She encouraged me to use herbal products.

At her suggestion, I used herbal shampoos and hair food, a skin toner, and the saffron (kesar) pack. When the saffron pack was introduced, Dr Shetty asked me to taste a bit. It was

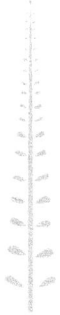

so yummy that till date, each time I apply it on my face, I am tempted to eat a little! The aroma keeps lingering around me. Every session made me better, not only externally but also within. After all, external beauty is a reflection of inner radiance!

Whatever Dr Shetty now asks me to do, I blindly follow. Such is the trust I repose in her!

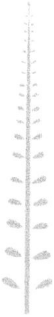

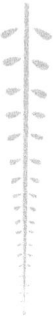

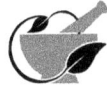

Acknowledgements

I would like to dedicate this book to my better half Jay, without whom this journey of mine would be incomplete, my sons Naveen and Ashwin for their encouragement, my daughter-in-law Sharanya for her support all throughout. I would also like to thank my friends and clients for their criticism and praises, and my mother who has nurtured me the natural way.

www.ingramcontent.com/pod-product-compliance
Lightning Source LLC
Chambersburg PA
CBHW071022280326
41935CB00011B/1461

9789384030438